Polyamory and Kink

by Jess Mahler

Dedicated to Dilip Numetor Amalia Chetana Waller.

For helping me see all this with new eyes.

(I warned you not to make me pick your pseudonym :P)

With thanks to:
Raven Kaldera, for doing it first.

My beta readers, Canageek and Daniel Cardoso,
for making this better than it would have been.

My Patrons, for believing in me.

Table of Contents

1 Introduction

Like it says on the front, this is a book about polyamory and kink. More specifically, this is a book about adding kink to your polyamorous relationships. My own background is in polyamory, so that's my focus in this (and most of my other writing). Folks doing other types of consensual nonmonogamy will also find parts of this book useful. As always, take what works, leave what doesn't.

This is not an 'intro to polyamory' book. I'm assuming readers have at least a basic working knowledge of what polyamory is and common polyam jargon. It is an 'intro to kink' book. Some folks reading this book will know nothing about kink. Maybe you aren't into kink yourself, but one of your partners is and you don't know what to expect. Maybe you have always wanted to get into kink but worried about how your partner(s) would react.

And some readers are likely kinksters who know WIITWD (What it is that we do) and can explain SSC (safe, sane and consensual) and its merits versus RACK (risk-aware consensual kink) backward and forwards. Let's not get you (or me!) started on the horror that is 50 Shades of Shit, right?

This book will likely be a very different experience depending on what you know about kink. If you are as vanilla as my favorite ice cream, you're about to learn a lot of stuff that may challenge you. If you've been in and around the Scene a few years, you will likely find a lot of the info here same-old, same-old.In order to make this book a good read for the greatest number of people, I'm putting all the 'what you should know about kink' stuff first. If you know your kink ABCs, you might want to skip some or all of the first section. If you are new to kink, I suggest reading everything and getting comfortable with it before adding kink to your relationships. Squicks are kinda like jealousy in a way. Unrecognized and undealt with they can ruin a relationship. Recognized and dealt with, they can be an occasional annoyance.

What are squicks, you ask?

That's why you need to keep reading. ;-)

1.1 Note on Terminology (For Everyone)

I'm going to try to define new terms as I introduce them, but there are a couple terms I want to introduce right away to head off any possible confusion. See, I'm using these terms a bit differently than usual in the Scene.

A top takes the active role in a scene.

Someone who's verse will sometimes top and sometimes bottom.

A bottom takes the passive role in the scene.

A dom likes to be in control.

A switch sometimes likes to be in control and sometimes likes to be controlled.

A sub likes to be controlled.

Most people in the Scene will generally agree with these definitions. BUT! will still use these words in a way that doesn't line up with the definitions. For instance, the default assumption in much of the Scene is that giving oral sex (often an active thing) is bottoming.

Similarly, many people conflate different roles. For instance, a top is assumed to be a dom and vice versa, or a sub is assumed to be a bottom.

Again, more on this later.

But if you are familiar with the Scene and my use of 'top' and 'bottom' seem odd, refer to these definitions.

Credit to CowhideMan, a true Old Guard, both in kink and leather, on Fetlife for suggesting 'verse' many years ago. 'Verse' is used among gay men for a man who likes to top and bottom sexually. CowhideMan proposed it for use in BDSM because folks tend to use 'switch' to refer to *both* someone who likes to top and bottom *and* someone who likes to control and be controlled. The confusion that caused was getting annoying to a lot of us in that particular Fet forum. As far as I know, his suggestion never gained much traction, but I'm using it, damnit!

1.2 Shout Out

I want to give a shout-out to *Power Circuits* by Raven Kaldera. *Power Circuits* was the first book about polyamory and kink and is well worth checking out if you are into power exchange. *Power Circuits* focuses specifically on D/s and especially M/s relationships. It's written for people with experience in D/s or M/s relationships who want to explore polyamory. If that is you, you may find *Power Circuits* very helpful in your explorations.

1.3 Who am I and Why am I Writing This Book?

My name, as it says on the cover, is Jess Mahler. I'm best known for my old polyamory blog, Polyamory on Purpose. These guides grew out of that blog. I've been 'doing' ethical nonmonogamy for nearly 20 years and polyamory for over 15 years. My first few nonmonogamous relationships are what we might euphemistically call 'learning experiences.' But with the help of folks like The Polyamorous Misanthrope and Fetlife's P&K group, I figured out what I was doing.

'P&K' by the way, stands for 'Polyamorous and Kinky.' I started experimenting with kink the same year I had my first experience with nonmonogamy. So I've actually got more experience with kink than with polyamory.

In polyamory, I lean towards group, communal relationships with high levels of entwinement. What I think of as the 'core' of my current polycule had plans underway to be living together within the next five years. In kink, I'm a dominant, top, bottom, masochist, sadist, rigger and rope slut. The only 'standard' kink identity I don't claim is submissive. I have submitted in the past but learned it hits some old trauma and puts me in a bad headspace. Plus I prefer being in charge. So I don't do it now. (If you are new to kink vocabulary, don't worry. I'll explain it all.)

So, I've lived at the intersection of polyamory and kink for nearly 2 decades now.

Like all the Polyamory on Purpose guides, I'm writing Polyamory & Kink because it's needed. The Venn diagram of polyamorous folks and kinky folks has a strong overlap. But there isn't much discussion about how that overlap works or how to navigate it. If you aren't familiar with that overlap, some aspects of kink, D/s in particular, can seem antithetical to polyamory.

So that's one reason and the main one. But the other reason is that unlike the other Polyamory on Purpose guides, I've actually had people ask for this one. So... that's who I am, why I'm writing this book, and why I think I have enough knowledge to write this book. That hits the high points, right?

Let's get to it.

1.4 Something in This Book Will Squick You

Everyone exploring kink for the first time should know two important terms:

1. Squick

2. YKINMK

Squick is a verb for feeling disturbed by something as well as a noun for something that disturbs you. It describes the reaction to a kink that you can't understand anyone doing.

For instance, scat play squicks me. My initial reaction every time I hear about scat play is "Ugh! Why?" Scat play is one of my squicks.[1]

YKINMK stands for "Your kink is not my kink". Scat play is not my kink. The thought of it is about the biggest turn off imaginable. But if it's your kink, that's okay. I don't need to like every kink. I don't even need to understand every kink.

I just need to not be an ass to people who have different kinks than I do.

Many people are going to be squicked by things in this book. That's okay. But you might find yourself rejecting and vilifying the things that squick you. That's not okay.

In polyamory, we talk about "leaning into" negative emotions. You don't ever need to do anything you don't want to in kink, and that 100% goes for anything that squicks you. But if you find yourself wanting to dismiss a kink as 'perverted', 'unnatural', or similar, it's time to lean into your squick. Just because you do not like it doesn't mean it's wrong for other people or that you can condemn other people for liking it. No one is the one and true arbiter of other people's kinks. YKINMK, and that's okay.

After all, food squicks many people. (Like, snails. OMG how the hell can anyone eat snails? *shudder*) But you don't go trying to shut down a restaurant that offers food you don't like. You eat somewhere else.

---

1   My nesting partner and bratty submissive is reading over my shoulder and suggesting scat play scenes we should try just to see me cringe.

2 What Is Kink?

Before we can talk about integrating polyamory and kink, we need to talk about *what is kink*. So... that's what we're going to do. We'll start with a basic discussion of what kink is (and is not). Then introduce different types of kink, some core concepts, and some basic health and safety for folks exploring kink.

2.1 Defining Kink

Anyone in online polyamory communities knows the endless discussions about how, exactly, to define polyamory.

For better or for worse, kink is harder to define than polyamory. But kinksters rarely try to define it.

Kinky folks tend to default to "BDSM", a far easier term to define.

BDSM is generally said to stand for

Bondage

Discipline

Sado-

Masochism

Some folks style it as Bondage, Dominance/submission, Sado-Masochism. In this version, the 's' does double-duty for submission and sadism. Bondage, D/s (sometimes called power exchange, though that also has a wider meaning), and SM are the three most common and well known kinky activities. However, kink encompasses more than the strict definition of BDSM.

For example, sensation play is a kinky activity that isn't

BDSM. Sensation play focuses on the use of various physical sensations to create pleasure. The best sensation play scene I know included food, scented candles, silk, satin, Wartenberg wheels, massage oils, feathers, and marbles. It used bondage, but didn't need to, involved no pain or discipline. The people in the scene were in a D/s relationship, but you could recreate it exactly without the D/s.

While this scene doesn't fall under the usual definition of BDSM, sensation play is part of kink. (And some readers are now realizing that they may be kinkier than they thought!)

So, what is kink?

The basic definition is usually something like 'an unusual sexual behavior.' Which is extremely vague, and not very useful. Daniel Cardoso commented to me that, "['kink'] presents itself as a kink (a wrinkle) in the supposedly flat surface of sexuality, which is supposedly determined by genitality. Kink usually shifts sexuality away from pure genitality, even when genitals are involved, they are so within a context that somehow does not toe the line from genital stimulation to orgasm."

To break that down out of academic-jargon, normally sex and sexuality is all about the genitals. Kink messes with that. Kink moves sex away from it's focus on genitals. Even when the genitals are involved in kink, they are used in a way that queers normal assumptions about sex and sexuality (for instance, the use of chastity devices).

This is, honestly, the best definition of kink I've come across.

There's just one problem...

2.1.1 It's Not All About Sex

While the popular view of kink is all about sex, the reality is... not. For many people, kink is part of (or in some cases, all of) their sex life. For others, kink (either in general or a specific inky activity) has nothing to do with sex.

For example, I've known many people for whom bondage is a form of meditation. For the rigger (person who ties the rope), complex bondage requires a kind of relaxed concentration similar to sitting zazen (a Buddhist meditation form). The rigger needs to maintain precise control of what their fingers are doing while maintaining a holistic awareness of the bottom's position and wellbeing, the state of the rope, and the progress of the tie.

For the rope bottom, bondage can be freeing and relaxing. A full-body tie can be like getting a full-body hug. I know several people who fall asleep best when in some form of bondage. Some autistic kinky folks say that a chest harness can be a good (and far less expensive!) substitute for a weighted blanket.

For all kinks that don't involve genitals (and possibly some that do), there are folks who enjoy them not as sexual activities, but just as a thing to do. This is important for non-kinky folks with a kinky partner to understand. There have been problems between kinky and non-kinky partners over this issue. A non-kinky partner might think an agreement not to have 'sex' with a new person without discussing it first covers all kinky stuff. But to their kinky partner bondage or a pup-play session at the local fetish party has nothing to do with sex. Drama incoming.

Both my pet and I enjoy being tied up. But we enjoy it for different reasons. Neither of which are sexual.

For me, bondage helps me get 'out of my head.' I am usually in a state of mild dissociation. The hypersensitivity that comes with being autistic makes being fully 'present' an overwhelming sensory hell. When I am tied up, the feel of the rope overwhelms the stuff going on around me. I can come out of the dissociation and be in my body for a while. This does have a sexual side for me, as it's hard to get into sex if you are experiencing high levels of anxiety or aren't 'in' your body. But sometimes I enjoy bondage for its own sake.

For my pet, bondage makes them feel safe—a common reaction. Another common sentiment is that a rope harness or body wrap feels like getting a 'full body hug.'

Of all people, polyam folks should be able to understand 'it's not all about sex.' Though, for many folks (myself included) kink is *mostly* about sex.

(This is also important for folks in kinky/'nilla monogamous relationships to understand, but that's a topic for another book.) Daniel and I spent some time talking his definition and non-sexual kink a bit, and I came up with this:

"I think kink can be a subset of sexuality AND be things that aren't sexual at all, and maybe we need two separate but related definitions to cover both of those, or maybe kink can (to steal ideas from Madeline Yergneau writing on a completely different topic[2]) be queering sexuality by *making* sexual things non-sexual, thus challenging the idea that what is sexual sometimes (including stuff involving genitals) is *always* sexual."

So, here's our final attempt at a definition of kink for today:

---

2   Madeline Yergeau, *Authoring Autism.*

> *Kink is queering the idea of what is sexual both by
> using nonsexual activities for sexual pleasure and by
> making normally-sexual activities (including kinky
> sexual activities) non-sexual.*

2.1.2 Kinky People Are Abuse Victims, Right?

Nope.

Not gonna lie, many kinky folks have been abused. You know why?

Because abuse is endemic in our society. There are lots of folks everywhere who have been abused. Including, if we are honest, in polyam communities. Kinky folks who are abuse survivors, like everyone else, have found ways of coping with the trauma we lived through.

However, kinky folks may be more open about our abuse and how it interacts with our activities. Joe who plays pick up basketball with you every week probably won't talk about the game helps him release the anger he's carrying from old abuse. That's too personal. But by the time most people comfortable telling you they are kinky, not much would be considered 'too personal.'

Think about it this way, what would you be more likely to tell a friend? That you were abused as a kid or that you get your ass beat for fun?

2.1.3 Hitting People Is Abuse

Actually, no.

If hitting people was abuse, then football, martial arts tournaments, fencing, boxing, MMA, hockey... (do I need to go on?) would all be abusive.

Hitting people in most jurisdictions legally counts as 'battery.' And while the activities I listed above are given a legal exception, BDSM is not. So a hit that would get you cheers sparring in the MMA ring can get you jail in BDSM. Thankfully, that rarely happens. But most folks who do pain play are aware of the legal risk they take.

When it comes to abuse, the much more fraught issue is control.

Psychologists, abuse support organizations, and survivors usually don't equate hitting with abuse. Instead, we define abuse as controlling or seeking to control someone's life and choices. I prefer to say that abuse is *denying someone their self-agency*. That's why hitting in a relationship is 'domestic violence'—to distinguish assault in a relationship from abuse. Most domestic violence involves abuse, but most abuse *doesn't* involve domestic violence. Hitting and other physical harm can be part of abuse. The physical attacks are a tool to keep someone under the abuser's control. But it's usually the last tool pulled out, after mental, emotional, verbal and often financial abuse has left the victim no avenue to resist or escape.

Dominance/submission (D/s) and other power exchange relationships are all about one person having control or power over the other person. What distinguishes D/s from abuse is consent. The sub wants to give up control to the Dom, the Dom is not *taking* control from the sub. And only within limits that everyone agrees to.

Similarly, what distinguishes pain play from domestic violence is consent. The bottom wants the pain and the top provides that pain within limits that everyone agrees to.

For polyamorous folks, this isn't a new idea—what's the difference between polyamory and cheating? *Consent.*

2.1.3.1 Abuse in D/s

Abuse does absolutely happen in relationships with kink. In fact, it is disturbing common. Not because kink is abusive but because abuse is common in every part of society.

While some folks like to think otherwise, the Scene's emphasis on negotiation and consent doesn't protect us from abusers. Worse, many abusers see submissive folks as easy targets. Having said that, it's important to note that not all victims are subs and not all abusers are Doms. Abusive subs do happen. And abusive switches. And abusive anything-you-can-think-ofs. In kink relationships that don't have a D/s element, abuse looks much like abuse in any relationship. In D/s relationships, it can be hard to tell the difference between consensual control and abuse. Especially from the outside.

However, there are some clear indications of when D/s has become abusive. In fact, everyone's 'favorite' romance series, 50 Shades of Grey, is a great example of abuse in D/s. We'll talk more about how to distinguish consensual and abusive D/s later.

2.1.3.2 So They Must be Mentally Ill, Right?

The Diagnostic and Statistical Manual of Mental Illness (DSM) does list sadism and masochism as mental illnesses. And 20 years ago the DSM listed homosexuality as a mental illness. The

The DSM is... well that's off topic. Let's just say it has it's, ah, *problems*. Anyway...

What a lot of people don't realize is that the sadism and masochism listings in the DSM have one important criterion. Sadism and masochism are only mental illnesses *if they are causing the patient significant distress*. If being a sadist is interfering with your life—you aren't eating right, or can't sleep, or it's cost you your job or something—it may qualify as a mental illness. May. (Sexual sadist, technically. The DSM doesn't consider anything unhealthy in being a non-sexual sadist or non-sexual masochist. Which, in my opinion, really says all you need to know about how valid *those* DSM listings are.)

But sadism and masochism, in and of themselves, aren't mental illnesses. They are an (admittedly uncommon) aspect of human variation. Humans are weird. That's just the way it is.

If you are squicked by pain play, that's okay, lots of people are. But society demonizes pain play a lot.[3] And it's really easy to pick up those demonizing ideas, like it being abuse or mental illness or evil or whatever your kool-aid of choice is and use it to justify your squick.

Please don't.

If you have *safety* concerns about how folks are playing—say you see someone doing impact play over the kidneys—speak up. Please! We want our play to be as safe as possible. But unless there is actual harm going on, please don't impose your squicks on your partners (or other folks, for that matter).

2.1.4 Kink Doesn't Exist in a Vacuum

The mundane world impacts kink, and vis-versa.

50 Shades of Grey has been the most visible example of this in recent years. Those books (which are hated for their inaccurate depiction of kink) have had a huge impact on the Scene. Partly by the number of new folks drawn to kink after reading those books. Partly in the way they have shaped vanilla society's view of kink.

In terms of individual relationships, we all bring things with us into kink. And those things impact our relationships with other people. D/s isn't the only kind of power imbalance in kink relationships—just the only one most of us have control over.

---

3   *Sexual* pain play, that is. For some reason beating people up (or watching people get beat up) in hockey, MMA and other contact sports is 100% okay to enjoy.

One person having a lot more money, a position in a local organization, more experience/knowledge, one person being out and the other not, and many other things can create power imbalances in relationships.

This isn't an exclusively kink thing, but I think it's important enough to get a mention. Anyone who deliberately uses this kind of power imbalance to control or influence their partners is an abuser and not someone you want to be in a relationship. Having this kind of power doesn't make a bad person and isn't something to feel guilty about. But if one of your partners says they are being harmed in someway because of these power imbalances, listen to them. It may be fine for *you* to always plan dates at your favorite kink club, but it's not so good for your partner if they are poor and can't afford the fees or if your black partner is hearing racist remarks from the dungeon monitors that you don't notice.

2.2 Introducing Kinks

Before we talk about different kinks, it's a good idea to cover fetishes. Fetishes are central to kink. Most kink play has a fetish embedded in it somewhere.

But what is a fetish? A fetish is something that a person takes pleasure from that is not usually considered pleasurable. Sometimes that's an 'in general' thing—few people enjoy being tied up, but some people to. Just liking being tied up can be part of a fetish, whether it's sexual or not. In other cases it's a sexual thing. Many people enjoy sharing food, but for some people sharing food can be a sexually pleasurable activity. Most kink involves sexual fetishes of one sort or another. And for some people kink is only about sexual fetishes. But not for everyone. You know the deal:

It's not all about the sex!

There are lots of different ways of categorizing fetishes. I tend to categorize fetishes as sensory, emotional, or sexual. Not all fetishes fall into these three categories, but most do. Which category a fetish falls into depends on what the focus of the fetish is.

Sensory fetishes are those where pleasure comes primarily from the 'five' senses. Common sensory fetishes are blindfolds, temperature play, massage, and pain play.

Emotional fetishes are when the pleasure comes primarily from the emotions the fetish elicits. These include humiliation play, control fetish, service fetish, fear play, and others.

Sexual fetishes involve the genitals, but aren't things most people will do, or even consider. Popular sexual fetishes are sounding, forced orgasms, fisting, edging, double penetration, are orgasm denial.

Note: many kinky activities connect with more than one fetish. For instance, for one person rope bondage may be a sensory fetish—they like the look and feel of rope. For another person rope bondage (and other types of bondage) are part of a control fetish. Similarly, spanking can be used as part of a pain fetish, a humiliation fetish, or a mix of the two. I've tried to put activities with the fetish they are *usually* associated with. But there are no hard and fast rules here.

That said, you can probably assume that someone who spends an hour or more on a complicated rope tie has a sensory-rope fetish.

Note two: Something doesn't need to be a sexual fetish to be, well, sexual. Many people are aroused by humiliation play. It is sexual for them—but it's not a sexual fetish. Remember: part of kink is making non-sexual things sexual.

So that's the general, let's take a look at some specifics. We're going to work off of BDSM here. The very fact that the acronym is so ubiquitous is proof of how common those kinks are. Go with what's been working.

2.2.1 Bondage

Bondage is all about being tied up. Usually literally, sometimes figuratively. The most common type of bondage is probably rope bondage, but handcuffs, cages, silk ties, scarves, and tape are all popular choices. From our types of kinks above, bondage generally falls under sensory or emotional.

The emotional side of bondage is easier to explain. Frankly, control fetish—enjoying having control or being controlled— ranks in the top 5 all-time popular fetishes. And bondage is a tool for physically controlling someone.

On the sensory side, the appeal of bondage can take many forms. A strict hogtie creates pain. A chest harness can feel like getting a hug. A cage can be a safe space, like a kinky version of a pillow fort. Breast bondage may trap blood in the breasts making them more sensitive. Some types of bondage can be literal works of art. (Don't believe me? Check out the rigger/photographer Garth Knight.) And for many folks bondage (both doing and receiving) can be meditative.

Bondage usually isn't a sexual fetish but can be. For instance, in rope bondage, a crotch rope means a rope that runs across the crotch, putting pressure on the genitals.

Common terms:

Rigger: Someone who ties people up with rope

Rope bottom/Rope slut/Rope bunny: Someone who likes being tied up with rope. (Some folks consider Rope slut or Rope bunny pejorative. Best to use only with folks who claim those terms for themselves.)

Common types of bondage:

Breast: Bondage that constrains the breasts in some fashion.

Hogtie: Both hands and ankles tied or cuffed together behind the back. A strict hogtie may include putting a gag or hood on the person bottoming and attaching that the tie, pulling their head back as well.

Harness: Rope or leather (usually) that wraps around the torso. Can be decorative or used as attachment points for further bondage.

Kinbaku/Shibari: A Japanese tradition of erotic bondage that has become popular in the West. Kinbaku is the traditional term, shibari a mistranslation that is common in English discussions of the art. Traditional kinbaku has a humiliation element that isn't common in the US. All versions of kinbaku I have seen have a heavy focus on being visually appealing.

Mummification: Full body bondage.

Vacuum beds: Use suction to trap a person between two pieces of latex with no way out. Risk of suffocation, never do alone.

Predicament bondage: Bondage that offers the bottom an either/or choice. Usually between types of pain but sometimes between pleasures. For instance, hands cuffed high enough you need to stand on tiptoes. Eventually, your calves start hurting. But if lower your body, your weight falls on your shoulders, which will start hurting.

Suspension: Bondage that holds the body fully or partly off the ground. Do not attempt alone.[4] Do not try to teach yourself.

Mental bondage: Coin flip whether this goes here or under D/ s. In mental bondage, the person bottoming holds *themself* in place. The person topping positions them, say, holding the headboard. Then the person bottoming needs to maintain that

4   With practice, self-suspension is possible. Don't try it without a lot of experience and someone on hand to help if necessary.

pose no matter what the top does. Sometimes the person bottoming is 'tied' up with string or something that will break if they aren't careful. Sometimes combined with predicament play.

2.2.2 Discipline or Dominance/Submission

Discipline refers to a power exchange relationship, of which the most common type is dominance and submission (D/s).[5]

Power exchange relationships are relationships where one person gives another power over them. Most power exchange relationships have a control fetish at their core. But the expression of control can take many forms and often mixes with other fetishes.

So what is a power exchange relationship?

In a D/s relationship, the submissive gives power to the dominant. The dominant has power over the submissive only as long as the submissive gives that power. The submissive determines *how much* power they give. There is a huge variety in D/s relationships. At one end, you have bedroom-only D/s with a number of hard and soft limits setting boundaries for what the dominant can do or order. At the other is 24/7 total power exchange (TPE) relationships where the dominant can, if they choose, control every aspect of the submissive's life. D/s is the most basic type of power exchange. Other power exchange relationships follow the same pattern as D/s, with some extra stuff added in.

As a shorthand, many kinky folks tend to refer to someone who receives power as a 'd-type' and the person who gives power as the s-type. For instance, 'It is important for the d-type to always remember their s-type's limits.' Power exchange relationships are written in the X/y format and sometimes people will talk about being the left (getting control) or right (giving control) side of the slash.

Of course, not everyone fits on one side of the slash and many people don't want to. People who can either give or receive power are called 'switches.' Some switches will switch within a single relationship—power flows back and forth between two people in whatever way suits them. Other people will always hold the same role in one relationship, but hold a different role in other relationships.

As with bisexuals, switches face erasure and prejudice. It isn't

5   In the past, D/s was an umbrella term for all power exchange relationships. These days it mainly refers to a specific type of power exchange, with 'power exchange' being the new umbrella term.

uncommon for subs, and particularly in my experience het male subs, to refuse to submit to a switch and insist a switch can't be a 'real dominant.' It rather reminds me of the whole 'gold star lesbian' bullshit.

Common types of power exchange:

Dominance/submission: your basic power exchange. One (or more) people give up control, one (or more) people take control

Master/slave: usually used for 24/7 TPE relationship or other power exchange where significant control is given up. Debates about the difference between sub and slave are endless.

Owner/pet: when the s-type has an animal persona. Pup play and pony play seem to be the most common, but kitten play is popular too.

Adult/little: when the s-type has a child or teen persona. Littles can range from infant through teen persona. Adults are usually called 'Mommy,' 'Dad,' or similar instead of more traditional PE titles. Hopefully goes without saying, but an adult having a child or teen *persona* doesn't make them any less an adult or any less capable of giving consent.

We'll be spending more time on power exchange that any other type of kink, so I'll introduce other common terms later.

2.2.3 Sado-Masochism (S&M)

Something I want to hammer home from the first: sadomasochism is *orthogonal* to power exchange. Many people, even in the Scene, equate being dominant with being a sadist and being masochist with being submissive. It doesn't work that way.

Having said that, let's talk about S&M.

Sado-Masochism is mostly a sensory fetish—a pain fetish. Sadists enjoy causing pain, masochists enjoy being in pain. Emotional pain is also a thing, however. So sometimes it can be an emotional fetish.

The idea of liking pain is hard for vanilla folks to grok, but I'll try to give a basic rundown. Bear with me, this is going to get science-y.

The body doesn't actually have any way to sense what we call 'pain.' Instead, the body has nerves that sense heat/cold, pressure, and some chemicals. When something hits your arm, the pressure nerves light up. The nerves send a signal to the brain saying how much pressure and how fast or slow the pressure increased. (This is why cuts from sharp knives often don't hurt immediately. They cut cleanly enough that there's no 'pressure' for these nerves to detect.) The brain then interprets the signal as a threat or not-a-threat. If it's interpreted as a threat, then the brain puts out an alarm. Essentially, our brain starts screaming 'Pain! Pain! PAINPAINPAINPAIN!!!'

Note: I'm not saying pain isn't real. Pain is very real. I'm saying that the cause of pain is more complicated than most people think.

Many things change whether or not the brain starts screaming 'Pain!' One of the best known is adrenaline. Adrenaline can shut down the body's alarm completely. This lets someone in a dangerous situation think and move without distraction.

This is why people in a fight may not feel pain until after the fight is over. They are harmed in the fight, but the adrenaline of fighting keeps the pain at bay. When they stop fighting and lose the adrenaline, the pain sets in.

So what does this have to do with masochism?

Some masochists don't have a literal pain fetish. We may not like pain any more than the next person. What some of us have is an extra setting in our brain. Sometimes, things that would *usually* cause a 'Pain!' alarm get interpreted as pleasure instead.

Which is why someone who can take a whip until they are bloody can be brought to tears by a stubbed toe. Different situations, interpreted by the brain differently.

Then you have adrenaline. Most masochists will experience at least a mild burst of adrenaline during a scene. In fact, many good sadists will deliberately construct a scene to increase the masochist's adrenaline levels. So that affects the pain sensations as well.

That covers part of it, but far from all. While many masochists don't experience pain in the same way, most of us do enjoy actual pain to one extent or another.

I know of two reasons for this. I expect there are others.

First, pain and pleasure mixed is a very different sensation than straight pain. Kind of like a mimosa is very different to drink than either orange juice or champagne on its own. So if you already have pleasure going (say, a vibrator or butt plug) and add pain to that (nipple clamps) it creates a mix of pain and pleasure that some folks really enjoy. Sometimes just for its own sake, sometimes for the secondary effects:

You know the endorphin high you can get from exercise?

Yeah, mixing pain and pleasure can give you that And that the adrenaline rush? Natural, safe, chemical-free high.

Not all masochists experience this, but many do.

Finally, for some masochists, the point isn't the pain, per se. The point is the emotions the pain brings. Many folks have used pain play reach to a point where they can release pent up, buried emotions. The pain play becomes a form of self-care for dealing with difficult-to-process emotions. While it isn't encouraged, per-se, everyone whose been around the Scene a while knows this happens. In an ideal world, this would involve people with training to combine pain play and emotional support/therapy. In the real world, it hopefully involves an experienced sadist or service top and at least one spotter to step in if there is a problem.[6]

From the sadist end...

At some point, you need to accept that some people enjoy fucked up things, and there's no clear reason for it. If I had to guess, I'd say it's related to how people instinctively lose sexual interest in familiar things. (Evolutionary biologists speculate that this prevents inbreeding. Your siblings are the most familiar people to you, so you won't be interested in them.) Taboo things are usually the most unfamiliar, and least subject to familiarity-blahs.

Every kinky sadist I know, including myself, has spent a lot of time wrestling with our desire to cause pain. For many of us, it flies in the face of everything we believe is good and right. Eventually, we usually come back to core ideas of kink—consent, mutual pleasure, and freedom to be ourselves without guilt or shame.

I don't know why I enjoy causing pain. I just do. But I will only do so when my partner wants it as much or more than I do.

Unfortunately, the Scene sometimes encourages a competitive aspect to masochism. It isn't uncommon for a masochist to brag about not having ever used a safeword or about the amount of pain they can take. Some sadists will boast about just how tough the masochist they play with is. This can lead to dangerous situations, as well as creating an unhealthy atmosphere for folks who aren't into pushing the pain limits.

Common terms:

---

6   We'll touch on this later, but sometimes instead of self-care, people use pain play as a way to *self-harm*. This is not healthy, nor is it accepted or supported in the Scene.

Pain slut: another term for a masochist. Has overtones of liking intense and/or extreme levels of pain. Often invoked competitively '...the biggest pain slut ever, you would not believe...'

Common types of S&M:

Impact play: pain caused by impact, what most folks unfamiliar with kink think of—whips, floggers, spanking, etc

______ Torture: when the pain is all about a specific body part, usually, but not always, tied to sex—breast torture, cock and ball torture, etc.

Needle play: using needles to cause pain, including needles inserted under the skin and left there for a while. Possible infection vector and other medical risks, training recommended.

Wax play: hot wax poured over the body, related to other types of temperature play. Often includes an aesthetic focus using different colors of wax.

2.2.4 Other Kinks

As mentioned earlier, there are a whole lot of ways to be kinky that don't fall under the BDSM acronym. Also a lot of stuff that many folks include in BDSM stuff that isn't necessarily part of the acronym. For what I hope will be a better reading experience, I'm putting a list, with brief descriptions, in the back of the book.

2.3 Important Kink Concepts

There are a few concepts from the Scene that it's important to know before discussing kink in any kind of depth. We will be spending a chunk of time on these—they will be important later.

2.3.1 Limits

Limits are one of the most important tools for healthy kink. Limits are just what the name says: *limits* on what a person is willing to or can't do, take part in, or have done to them. Some limits are physical—someone with bad knees can't kneel for a long time. Even if they could endure the pain, they would be harmed by it. If they didn't care about *that*, sooner or later their body would give out. Some limits are psychological, the result of phobias, trauma, or plain old self-preservation. Most limits are choices, things a person can do or endure, but doesn't want to.

Whatever the basis of the limit—physical limit, psychological limit, or limit by preference—limits are the boundaries of consent. They should always be respected as such. To willingly or intentionally violate a person's limits is to violate their consent and break their trust. I shouldn't need to explain why this is a bad thing.

Similarly, never pressure someone to change their limits, shame them over their limits, or otherwise coerce them to change their limits.

Kinky folks tend to talk about two kinds of limits: hard limits and soft limits.

Hard limits are the 'No, never, don't ask!' of the kinky world. It's something you will not do, period.

Soft limits are a kind of 'No for now.' Soft limits are still limits. Other people don't get to pressure you about them or ignore a limit because they think you'll like it or any shit like that. Soft limit means *you* are leaving the possibility open to try this in the future. Some soft limits are conditional. For instance, many kinky activities can be dangerous if not done right. A bottom might have a soft limit on, say needle play, even though they really like needle play. They won't do needle play until their inexperienced partner gets lessons from an expert. Or a soft limit might be circumstantial, 'No penetration without a barrier method.' They will do penetration, but only under specific circumstances.

Many people new to kink might have a giant list of soft limits, things they are curious about but don't feel safe or comfortable trying. Over time many of those soft limits will be explored in a safe and comfortable setting. Then they usually become hard limits (if the person doesn't like it) or a new fetish (if they do).

Because it's a consent thing, discussion of limits happens early before any kinky stuff happens. Some folks tell each other their limits as part of a casual conversation. But there is so *much* in the realm of kink that it's easy to forget some of it. Which is why BDSM checklists are circulating the internet.

Each person takes one copy of a checklist and marks of each item. Most checklists have options for 'like,' 'haven't tried,' 'soft limit' and 'hard limit.'

Then potential play partners compare their lists, which can run to several pages. If they have any limits they have that aren't mentioned on the lists, they add them.

The nice thing about these lists is you can keep them with you, so you can refer back if you need to. You can use lists to refresh your memory or for inspiration. Sometimes a list can be a big help in coming up with a new scene or activity to try.

The *problem* with these lists is they assume everyone fits on one side of the slash. You are expected to fill them out *either* as a top/d-type *or* as a bottom/s-type. This can be frustrating to lots of folks who switch, are verse, or don't fit the top=d-type stereotype.

2.3.2 Negotiation

Negotiation is a key process to most any kinky stuff. And a major hurdle in vanilla folks understanding kinky relationships.

See, negotiation means something different in kink.

Since I hate reinventing the wheel, here's how I explained it in *Safer Sex for the Non-Monogamous*:

> Folks who aren't familiar with kink will probably be choking a bit on 'negotiation.' To many people, negotiation implies compromise and agreeing to do something you don't want to do so you can get what you want.
>
> That's not the way consent negotiations are meant to be done. The idea of a consent negotiation isn't to negotiate against your connection to get what you want. It's to negotiate with your connection to get the experience that will be best for both of you.

Kinky negotiations start by laying out what you are into, what you aren't into but will enjoy if your partner(s) are into, and what you won't do. Like building a plate from a buffet, you and your partner go through the things everyone is into or ok with. Together you decide which of those things you will include in your scene and/or relationship. If there is something you are both into, it goes on the plate. If there is something you are into and your partner is okay with, maybe a little bit of that goes on the plate. (And vis versa.)

Often something you are really into is a limit (hard or soft) for someone else. The negotiation process is how you find these preference-clashes and decide how to deal with it. Most often 'decide how to deal with it' means you don't include X thing in the scene or relationship.

Sometimes, especially when discussing relationships, it means you have a fundamental incompatibility. For instance, two d-types who are looking for a power exchange relationship have a problem. These relationships either won't work or will only work with great difficulty and sacrifice. Usually, at that point, everyone agrees that this isn't going to work. But sometimes it's worth trying. Especially if you share other kinks you want to explore together.

2.3.2.1 Relationships vs Scenes

Just a quick note—negotiation works for both relationships *and* scenes. You can negotiate the big stuff at the beginning of a relationship. Stuff like PDAs, safer sex boundaries, whether to do D/s bedroom only, 24/7, or not at all, etc. Then you negotiation specific things for a given scene. Stuff like whether the scene will include bondage, what kind of bondage, will it be a role play scene, etc.

2.3.3 SSC/RACK

There are a couple different philosophical approaches to ethics in kink. The two most common are SSC and RACK. A newer idea that is starting to gain traction is the 4Cs.[7]

SCC stands for 'safe, sane, and consensual.' RACK stands for 'risk-aware consensual kink.'

There are two big differences between the two philosophies. One that most people immediately notice, the other that many people miss.

The obvious difference is the approach to safety. SSC requires that kink play be safe, or as safe as the participants can possibly make it. (After all, you can't be completely safe just crossing the street!)

RACK is okay with risk. Folks who engage in edge play and extreme pain play, as well as other kinks with a higher potential for accidental harm, are more likely to espouse RACK. RACK requires that everyone involved be aware of the risks they take and consent to those risks.

But not everyone who adopts a RACK philosophy is doing risky kink. Some RACK folks feel that since it is impossible to be 100% safe, it's important to emphasize risk awareness—no matter how big or little that risk is.

The other difference that doesn't get as much notice is that

---

7   The 4Cs were first laid out in the paper "From 'SSC' and 'RACK' to the '4Cs': Introducing a New Framework for Negotiating BDSM Participation."

Williams, D & Thomas, Jeremy & Prior, Emily & Christensen, M. Candace. (2014). From "SSC" and "RACK" to the "4Cs" : Introducing a New Framework for Negotiating BDSM Participation. Electronic Journal of Human Sexuality. 17.

RACK doesn't have equivalent to SSCs 'sane.' Sane was included (in fact some sources say SSC itself was developed) as a response to the common view that sadomasochism (and by extension all kink/BDSM practices) was a mental illness and abusive. But as kink has gained broader acceptance, some problems with the word have come to the fore.

Many RACK folks argue that including 'sane' in SSC implies that some kinks are not sane. The 'sane,' then, is ableist and kink-shaming. Another problem is the 'sane' of SSC can become exclusionary to people with mental illness. Finally, as the authors of the 4Cs point out, 'sane' is a legal term and maybe we shouldn't be dragging legal terminology into WIITWD. (Unless, of course, that's your kink.)

Not all, or even most, SSC people intend to exclude people with mental illness. But it does happen. Even when it doesn't happen, stigma against mental illness is a real problem. Some folks who deal with mental illness will shy away from any group that has 'sane' as one of their requirements.

Yes, group.

SCC and RACK started as philosophies for individual kinksters. Over time, many play groups, dungeons, and munches have chosen one or the other philosophy to be part of their group's rules. Folks who join a RACK group don't need to embrace RACK themselves. SSC folks are welcome as long as they follow the group's rules. And the reverse is true as well.

Personally, I lean towards RACK, both as someone who believes complete safety it an unrealistic goal and as someone who has struggled with mental illness. I realize that my bias is coming through in this section. If I can, I'll fix that in revisions, but if not, I can at least acknowledge that I have this bias.

The 4Cs are consent, communication, caring, and caution. It is, as I said, a new approach that seeks to address the same needs as SSC and RACK while addressing some of the gaps. Consent, obviously, is in all three terms, and caution here stands in as an alternative to 'safe' and 'risk-aware.' The creators of the 4Cs note that what is risky has come to be defined not by the people engaging in kink, but by medical and academic professionals. This is creating the same problem that the RACK folks originally objected to in SSC—that some kinks are getting labeled as 'too risky.' People who engage in them are being excluded from the Scene based on the judgments of non-kinksters.

So the authors of 4Cs propose caution as an alternative.

Caution can be self-defined. Participants can decide for themselves what level of caution is best for their comfort/needs.

The new terms here are caring and communication. In SSC and RACK, communication is usually addressed as a subheading of consent. Here it is its own heading, a key piece of kink play in its own right. The authors focus on caring during negotiations—that it is not enough to negotiate for what you want and need. You need to negotiate with care in mind for your partner and their wants/needs. Caring also applies during the scene and, of course, to aftercare, but caring in that sense is usually (rightly or wrongly) seen as the province of the top/dom. In negotiations and more general interactions, caring is important for everyone.

I have heard mention of a fourth approach, PRISM, on and off over the past few years. I have never heard details of it, and don't recall the general descriptions I did see. Unfortunately, I haven't been able to find any publicly available discussion of it. I'm assuming it isn't very widespread or well known.

2.3.3.1 BORK

In the course of writing this book, I learned about BORK from Michael Vogel. BORK is 'balls out risky kink'. Michael V. described it as '... no limits, no safety. It's the opposite of SSC and RACK basically.' It's not common (or I would have heard of it before). And it's not generally supported in the Scene. I suppose BORK folks are the kink equivalent of BASE jumpers. Not something I'd ever want to be involved in, but if it's what the people involved want... well, not my business to judge.

2.3.4 Safeword

Safewords are a common safety and consent tool in kink.

A safeword is a word that the participants agree to use if a problem occurs and they need to stop the scene. A safeword is a word that you wouldn't normally say. Some people choose safewords that are things they dislike, but generally, it's a neutral word that wouldn't come up in conversation. 'Asparagus' is a popular joke safeword. There was a t-shirt that was briefly meme'd in kink spaces. As best I recall, it read "Sometimes 'No' means 'no.' Sometimes 'Asparagus' means 'no.' "

Bottoms and s-types use safewords most often, but tops and d-types can and do safeword as well.

There are several reasons to use a safeword during a scene or in a relationship.

1. In a roleplay scene, having a safeword allows the bottom to

say things like 'no, stop, don't!' in their roleplay character and the top knows everything is okay, it's part of the game. The bottom can fully enjoy the role while knowing that they can stop it in an instant with their safeword.

2. Allows begging/pleading to be part of a scene. Sometimes a person finds themself saying 'stop' or 'no.' But it's a reflex and they don't want things to stop. Trying to control themself to not say it keeps them from relaxing and enjoying the scene. Having a safeword lets them relax and say whatever they need to. If they need to stop the scene, they can safeword and know the person they are playing with will understand.

3. Not being able to say 'no' or 'stop.' Many people might not be able to say 'no' or 'stop' in mid-scene. They might be deep in subspace, they might be borderline non-verbal, they might be gagged...

And that leads into our next point. A safeword can be anything. It can be a hand sign, a bell someone can drop or ring, or any number of signals that don't necessarily involve your voice.

Most folks talk about safewords in a scene and as something that s-types and/or bottoms use. But safewords can be used at any time, and anyone can use them. A d-type or top can safeword out of a scene if they need to, and safewords can be used in social situations or any place else. Sometimes it helps to have a way to say 'get me out of here' so your partner(s) know you are serious.

The main thing about safewords is they are for when you don't have time or ability for in-depth communication. *Not* to replace communication.

So if someone safewords, always follow up later. Ideally, everyone involved should understand what happened, why, and what to do if it happens again. Sometimes you can't get that. Sometimes the person who safeworded doesn't understand why they needed to. That's okay. But as much understanding as possible is important.

Note, I don't say 'how to prevent it from happening again.' Some things you can prevent, and should. But things like a rope tightening and causing numbness, or a flashback being triggered, aren't things you can 100% avoid. Do what you can to avoid them, but know that they may happen again. You should either have a plan for how to handle it (which can include safeword and stop the scene') or avoid that type of play until you do have a plan.

Safewords also have accessibility uses. Someone with PTSD may not feel safe saying 'no,' possibly to the point of having an anxiety or panic attack. Someone with autism may become nonverbal under intense sensation. And there are many reasons that someone might use safewords, in a scene, in vanilla sex, or in daily life.

2.3.4.1 Stoplight System

The best-known safeword within the Scene is actually three safewords—red, yellow and green.

The stoplight system uses color codes that allow the d-type and/or top to check in during a scene and make sure that everything is okay. Green means everything is good, keep going. Yellow is used in two different ways. It can mean that the bottom needs the scene/activity to slow down a bit, or that they need to stop and talk before resuming play. Red means stop everything, the scene is over.

If you play in a public kink-friendly space, expect most folks there to know this system and respect it.

Some clubs/groups might require kinksters use the stoplight system so Dungeon Monitors can recognize when someone is using a safeword.

Variations on the stoplight system are common. Some folks add extra colors for other things they might want to communicate when they can't string a full sentence together. I've heard of folks with PTSD using a specific color to mean they are having a flashback or panic attack. Lots of folks apply their own slightly different meaning to 'red' or 'yellow.' There are lots of other variations.

One advantage of the stoplight system is that most of the world uses stoplights these days with red/yellow/green lights meaning all the same thing. So most folks don't have trouble remembering 'hey, what does green mean?' We all know green means go, even when half out of minds with pleasure. And the opposite for red.

2.3.5 Good Pain and Bad Pain

Not as universal as the other concepts in this section, but still good to know. Which it comes to pain play, there is 'good pain' and 'bad pain.' (This is primarily about masochists but folks who aren't masochists experience this too.)

What is good pain and what is bad pain will be different for each and depending on their relationship on pain.

In general, there are three ways to view whether pain is good or bad:

Is it pleasurable or unpleasurable? This is a big thing for many masochists, they want pleasurable pain and don't want unpleasurable pain.

Is it superficial or harmful? Most of us can tell the difference between the feeling of an ouchy bruise or a bone bruise. Between a scratch and a deep cut. Between the burn of pushing our limits in exercise and a strained muscle. Not all harmful stuff is painful and not all harmful pain is recognizable. But mostly it is. For the majority of folks doing pain play, and everyone not trying to do pain play, pain that indicates harm is bad pain. Non-harm pain may or may not be good pain, depending on what you are going for.

Is it intentional or unintentional? I've seen and heard more scenes go bad from unintentional pain than almost anything else. The danger with unintentional pain is that the bottom may not realize it's unintentional and not speak up, and the top may not realize it's happening. Sometimes, this can just mess with the flow of the scene. Sometimes it is dangerous, as that unintentional pain may be unrecognized harmful pain.

Being aware of what is good pain and what is bad pain is an important part of healthy kink. For the bottom, this means speaking up or safewording if they recognize a pain as bad pain. For the top, this means checking on how the bottom feels, not just in general, but about specific things. I.e., do the cuffs hurt? How are your knees feeling? etc.

2.3.6 Hurt vs Harm

Related to good pain and bad pain, many kinky folks distinguish between hurt and harm. Hurt is pain. It's a physical (or emotional) sensation. But some things that hurt are good for you. Or at least neutral. Growing pains hurt. Having a dislocated shoulder fixed hurts. Facing the ways you screwed up and committing to doing better in the future hurts. Getting your ass flogged hurts.

But those things don't cause *harm*. In kink, we don't want *harm* but sometimes we want *hurt*. Harm is damage. How much damage a vague thing. After all, a bruise is caused by bleeding under the skin, but most folks don't consider a small bruise damage. On the other hand, bruised *kidneys* are harm, not just hurt.

Anyway, that's the basic idea. Hurt is a neutral concept that can be good or bad depending on the context. Harm is bad and should be avoided. Everyone will have a different idea of what *exactly* 'harm' is, so, ya know, communication.

2.3.7 Aftercare

Kink can be intense, right? I mean you don't need to know anything about kink to know that getting whipped is an intense experience. Sometimes, when a scene is finished, one or more participants will need help to recover.

In kinky communities, that 'help' is called 'aftercare.'

Everyone will have different aftercare needs. Needs can also vary with what type of scene you had. However, some needs are pretty common:

Water and food. An intense scene will take a lot of energy and can leave a person dehydrated (sweat, panting, etc). So a drink and high energy food are a common part of aftercare. Many folks who play in public will carry water bottles and oranges or chocolate bars with them for after the scene. Some clubs and dungeons will also have bottled water and snacks available for people who need them.

Pain relief. Advil, topical pain creams, massage, ice packs, are all common parts of aftercare. Unsurprisingly, folks who do pain play need them most often, but you can strain a muscle in vanilla sex or, hell, tripping over the chair someone forgot to push in. Being in one position for a long time can result in soreness, or someone may have an old injury or chronic pain condition that flares up. So stuff for pain is a pretty common part of aftercare kits, even if many people don't expect to need it.

Emotional/mental care. Cuddles, verbal reassurance, some quiet/low sensory space/time, pillow fort to hide in. There are several ways a kink scene can put someone in an altered mental or emotional state. Some scenes, such as humiliation play, that's kind of the point. But also scenes that bring on sub- or dom-space (more on those later), any form of punishment scene, many role play scenes (interrogation scene comes to mind), and others. And then there the way non-kink issues can impact kink. Someone who is hypersensitive or has recent sexual trauma is likely to need this care frequently.

Many people keep a box or bag of aftercare supplies on hand when they are doing a scene.

Sometimes people don't need aftercare.

Sometimes the aftercare people need doesn't look like

aftercare. I spoke with a submissive once who said she didn't need aftercare, she needed to go right back to the normal routine of serving her dom. So after a scene, she'd bring him a drink and do whatever else he told her. I would argue that she did need aftercare. She said she *needed* to go right back to the normal routine. That routine was her aftercare. It was, as she said, upsetting for her to cuddle or get cared for after a scene. I doubt that it was generally upsetting to her to have her husband/dom cuddle with her. More likely she did have needs for care after the scene. The return to normalcy gave her what she needed to cope with the emotions the scene created. And her dom, credit to him, gave her that.

Most of the time, folks need aftercare when an intense scene ends. And most of the time when people talk about aftercare, they are talking about the bottom or sub needing aftercare.

But neither of those are necessarily the case. In my case, I will often need care the day after an intense topping scene. After the scene, I'm focused on taking care of the person I played with and enjoying the afterglow of a good scene. But by the next morning, I tend to crash, hard.

If I'm topping and a scene goes bad, I may need aftercare sooner. I've got enough trauma in my background that a bad scene can stir up a lot of shit and leave me a wreck. Luckily, that doesn't happen often.

If both the top and the bottom can need aftercare, unless you have other people helping out,[8] someone needs to come first.

As a general rule, the bottom should get aftercare first, because they are the one on the receiving end of the scene. But use your own judgment. If you bottom and only need to rest a bit, but your top needs to be held and reassured that you didn't take the thing they said in your humiliation scene personally and they know you love them, etc, then it's okay to give them what they need first.

2.4 Not Everything Is Okay

YKIMK and that's okay—except when it's not.

Look, every kink is 'okay' means people aren't in control of their kinks and no one should be shamed or blamed for the things that turn them on. That doesn't mean that kinky *activities* are never problematic or toxic. Consent is an obvious limit on

---

8   Or even if you have, since most folks do best with aftercare from their play partner.

this—you can have a noncon kink. It still isn't okay to ignore consent. Enjoy all the noncon erotic novels you like. Fiction is fiction—but that doesn't belong in real life.

Similarly, no shame if you kink on role play as a slave owner in the antebellum South. But given the harm that bit of history caused, you should think real hard before you act out that kink. (Especially if you are a white American).

No one should be shamed or blamed for *having a kink*. But harm isn't just physical. If acting out your kink will cause harm, that's probably not something you should be doing.

If acting out your kink will recreate a historical harm, that's something you should think long and hard before doing. Especially if the historical harm still has traumatic impact today. At minimum, you should warn any people involved in or witnessing the scene. They need a chance to opt-out.

3 NonMonogamy in Kink

3.1 Lean the Fuck In

NonMonogamy is actually extremely common in the Scene. For instance, cuckolding/cuckqueening is a common kink that is *based* on being nonmonogamous. However, nonmonogamy in the Scene is very different from polyamory. Polyamory and nonmonogamy in the Scene are based on different premises.

In fact, nonmonogamy in the Scene takes several forms, each of them with their own premise. For instance (and *lean in* here), cucking is based on the idea that your partner needing or wanting another partner is *humiliating*. The cucks 'failure' as a sexual partner is the 'justification' for their partner having other sexual partners.

Even for me, 15 years polyam and longer in kink, that one makes me uncomfortable. Which is why I started with it. *Lean in.* Leave the judgment at the door. Kinky people do nonmonogamy different than polyamorous folks, but it's what they choose. (Yes, including the cuck. In fact, I know several relationships where the cuck initiated the dynamic.)

The other forms of nonmonogamy in kink are less... blatantly offensive to polyamorous sensibilities. But they do tend to strike many polyam folks as *wrong*. Egalitarianism is at the basis of most approaches to polyamory. Any hierarchy-based approach to nonmonogamy (as in power exchange relationships) is going to be very different. So are relationships *kinking* negative cultural assumptions about nonmonogamy (as in cucking). If you want to connect with kinky folks, you need to be ready to lean in to very different approaches to nonmonogamy.

I'm not saying you should change *your* approach to nonmonogamy. If polyamory makes you happy, stick with it! (I certainly have.) But polyamory ain't the only way to do ethical nonmonogamy. And if you haven't figured that out by now, you better get a handle on it soon.

3.2 Because Incompatibility Happens

Okay, we've introduced the type of kinky nonmonogamy polyamorous readers are most likely to choke on. Let's go easy and spend some time on something familiar. Sexual incompatibility has brought many people to polyamory over the years. Well, incompatibility in kink is also a thing. Some folks can't do sex without kink. Others need kink outside of sex. If a vanilla and a kinky person are in a relationship, that can be a big incompatibility. People in relationships can also have incompatible kinks—for instance two s-types or two d-types in a relationship. Opening the relationship is one way to address the incompatibility.

Not everyone agrees on when a relationship is nonmonogamous. Kink, you will recall is not all about sex, but most folks define monogamy and nonmonogamy by sex. For instance, a masochist married to a vanilla person may have a regular kink partner for pain play, but only have sex with their spouse. They still consider themselves monogamous, because there is no sex between the masochist and their play partner. But another couple in the same situation might consider it nonmonogamy.

Of course, if there is sex just about everyone considers it nonmonogamy.

3.3 NonMonogamy in Power Exchange

Most nonmonogamy in the Scene is probably connected to power exchange relationships. We'll look into several common or recognized structures for nonmonogamous power exchange later. Right now, you need to wrap your head around one thing: any nonmonogamous power exchange has a baked-in hierarchy.

A power exchange relationship is, by definition, hierarchical. The d-type has control over some things the s-type does. However, power exchange hierarchy is different from polyamory hierarchy.

In the primary/secondary prescriptive hierarchies, the

hierarchy is between relationships. If I want to date someone with a prescriptive primary/secondary hierarchy, I am part of that hierarchy. My relationship with them will always be 'secondary.' That is a box the other relationship is putting my relationship in.

In power exchange hierarchies, the hierarchy is between people. If I want to date someone in a power exchange hierarchy, I am not part of that hierarchy. That hierarchy says nothing about what my relationship with my partner is or may become.

That doesn't mean that a power exchange hierarchy wouldn't affect my relationship with someone. But for the most part, no more than any relationship will. If my partner needs to be home by 8pm weeknights, it doesn't matter to me if it's because their dom made that a rule or because they have to put the kids to bed. The impact on my relationship with them is the same.

Sometimes a power exchange hierarchy will have more severe and direct impacts. We'll look at that, and how to navigate it, later.

But check the assumptions, okay?

3.4 NonMonogamy as a Kink

Sometimes, as with cucking, nonmonogamy is the kink. NonMonogamy isn't usually a kink on its own but is usually found in combination with other kinks. For instance, cucking combines nonmonogamy, humiliation, and exhibitionism/voyeurism. A Master 'giving' her slave to someone else to use sexually is combining control kink with nonmonogamy.

In these cases, the nonmonogamy aspect usually functions as an open relationship. Casual or FWB sexual encounters outside the main relationship while strong emotional ties are kept within the main relationship. However, sometimes a committed group relationship will develop. For instance, a Dominant ordering two subs to have sex with each other can be casual on the part of the subs. But it can evolve into a committed triad depending on the desires, limits, and needs of the people involved.

3.5 Take Some Time to Process

We're going to take a break from kinky nonmonogamy for a bit to talk about mixing general kinks with polyamory. I know a lot of polyam folks will find this section on kinky nonmonogamy very challenging. Take this subject change as a chance to process and get used to some of the new ideas I just threw at you. We'll be coming back to them, especially nonmonogamous power exchange, in a bit.

4 Kink and Polyamory?

As you can see, kink and polyamory have all the ingredients for a major culture clash. Bringing kink assumptions into polyamory, or polyamorous assumptions into kink, is a recipe for drama. That isn't to say that polyamory and kink can't work together. They can, beautifully. But, there can be misunderstandings and miscommunications if you aren't careful.

However, I want to point out three more differences between polyamory and kink. In particular, some areas where one can be more problematic than the other:

Polyam communities, in general, are making an effort to be inclusive of folks of all genders. Many leaders in the polyamory communities (in fact the founders of polyamory communities) were women. As a non-binary person, people make an effort to respect my gender, and writings will generally be inclusive of all genders. Folks fall on their faces from not knowing how to be inclusive, but the effort is there. There is a similar, and markedly less successful, effort to be inclusive of LGBT and PoC.

In many kinky spaces, gender inclusion is... not so much. Sexism is alive and well in the Scene and along with that comes the default to the gender binary. Kink does better than polyamory (though still not great) in making space for gender-binary LGBT folks.

From what I've seen neither group has many loud-and-proud racists—or any patience for them. But tokenism and fetishizing of PoC is alive and well, along with the usual structural issues.

Another big difference is the handling of jealousy. Talk of jealousy and jealousy management in kink spaces, even among non-mono kinky folks, is rare. Occasionally you will see someone post in a forum about their struggle with jealousy. A good quarter of the responses will be something like, 'It's your D-types right to take another s-type if they want. If you don't like it, get out.' Most responses are more supportive, but the gist is still 'If you can't handle your jealousy, you shouldn't be in a non-mono relationship.' There will be some generally helpful replies, but they are in the distinct minority.

In contrast, it's hard to find any polyam stuff that isn't about managing jealousy and the emotional side of polyam relationships. That's the whole reason I started the Polyamory on Purpose blog—I wanted something different. We don't shut up about jealousy, we just plain don't.

Finally, kink doesn't have the evangelical attitude common to many polyamorous communities. Kink groups will usually welcome newcomers, but there is no general effort to convert people to kink; no idea that kink is better or more 'enlightened' than vanilla. A kinky person will likely try to introduce a vanilla partner to kink. They will not tell a vanilla person online that vanilla is inherently toxic and unethical.[9]

So yeah, the culture-shock of a polyam and kinky nonmonogamous person getting together is real.

A monogamous kinky person exploring polyamory face all challenges that any monogamous person has. But they will usually be familiar with nonmonogamy. Maybe have seen some nonmonogamous relationships in action.

Having covered that, let's get to actually putting polyamory and kink together. Part one here is about kink in general, whether or not power exchange is involved. After this section, we'll be taking an in-depth look at power exchange. Then how to integrate power exchange and polyamory.

4.1 Play to Your Strengths

For all the potential challenges, kink and polyamory have a fair bit in common. Both have a strong focus on communication and consent. Both encourage people to lay out their own needs and desires in a relationship. If you are following best practices for either, you have ditched mainstream assumptions about what a relationship looks like.

If you want to integrate kink into your polyamory, start with

---

9   If you haven't been aware of this happening in polyamory, lucky you. I've been hearing horror stories—and trying to help recovery—from mono folks for years. Be more aware, and put a stop to this shit.

the things they share.

4.1.1 Building a Bespoke Relationship

Leave the assumptions at the door. The assumptions about what kink is, about how relationships should work. *And* the assumptions that words (hierarchy comes to mind) mean the same thing to you as they do your partners. Be prepared to start with a clean slate.

4.1.2 Communicate, Communicate, Communicate

Look, for kinksters and polyam folks this should go without saying. It's the corollary to ditching the assumptions. You need to talk. And not just your usual new relationship conversations—what everyone needs, wants, etc. You need to understand each other's perspectives. How each of you views polyam and kink. How you define a relationship. Your relationship history in kink or polyamory and how it impacts your view of relationships and what you expect from your partner(s). Boundaries vs rules vs limits and how each of you views them, how to integrate one (or more!) into your relationship(s). The different safer sex risks involved in different kinds of sex and different kinds of kink.

Some questions to consider:

Will it be egalitarian polyam or will there be a hierarchy? What kind of hierarchy?

Kink only in sex? Or in other areas of life/relationship?

How will safer sex be handled?

Is everyone aware of the risks they will be taking with the types of kink?

Will power exchange be a factor and how will it affect people outside the exchange?

Just... talk. A lot.

4.1.3 Consent Isn't as Simple as You Think

This should be relationships 101. It isn't.

What does consent mean? Does consent mean 'enthusiastic consent?' Consent-as-negotiation? Consent-as-process? 'No means no?' There have been many ways of defining and framing consent over the years. In kink, the focus is usually on consent-as-negotiation. Enthusiastic consent is popular in polyam circles but has its detractors.[10] Consent-as-process is becoming common.

Make sure everyone is on the same page about what consent means.

Every relationship should have this discussion.

Specific to kink and polyamory, make sure everyone consents to the *types of relationship you are building*.

Hopefully, if you did the communication bit, everyone wants to build the same type of relationship.

But chances are, you missed something. It's impossible to catch all our assumptions, to communicate everything, especially the first time. That's okay.

If something comes up that wasn't discussed before, take a step back.

Don't accuse, and don't get defensive. If someone else's actions or assumptions surprised you, you can say, "Hey, I think we missed this in our discussions. Can we talk about it?"

If your actions or assumptions surprise someone else, realize that they didn't have a chance to consent to this. And make time to talk about it as soon as possible.

Sometimes, these things can feel like a betrayal or an ambush. If you need to, it's okay to step back, take some time to process your emotions, and discuss it later. You can come to the discussion ready to work with your partner, and not conflict with them.

4.1.3.1 Consent as Negotiation vs Consent as Process

I introduced consent-as-negotiation back in the first chapter but didn't get into consent-as-process. I'm going to put my descriptions of consent-as-process and consent-as-negotiation from *Safer Sex for the Non-Monogamous* together here. This way you and your partner(s) can easily compare and discuss them.

Consent as process:

Society and culture tend to teach consent as a thing or an event. It goes something like this:

Teens are (hopefully) told not to have sex unless their connection gives consent.

10 For my issues with enthusiastic consent, check out *Safer Sex for the Non-Monogamous*.

So when they want to have sex, teens ask some theoretically sexy version of "will you have sex with me?"

If the person they ask says yes, consent has been given, no further thought is given to consent, they have sex.

But that's not healthy consent. It's a model of consent that assumes everything will stay as it was the moment consent was given or withheld and that both people have the same idea of what agreeing to 'sex' means. It's also an all-or-nothing model of consent. Either you consent to sex or you don't. And this violates the requirement that healthy consent be informed.

Let's look at consent as a process.

Ace asks Beth is he can go down on her. This is 1) more specific in what consented to and 2) easier to make into verbal foreplay.

Beth agrees, but after a few minutes tells Ace to stop and kiss her.

Ace agrees and asks Beth to touch him. Beth does.

Throughout their time together, they continue communicating wants and needs. The process of consent continues until they are mutually finished or one of them withdraws consent and they stop.

Threesomes and moresomes make consent-as-a-process somewhat more complicated, but still doable. Just be sure to check in before you engage with someone and to check in regularly after that.

Consent as negotiation:

Folks who aren't familiar with kink will probably be choking a bit on 'negotiation.' To many people, negotiation implies compromise and agreeing to do something you don't want to do so you can get what you want.

That's not the way consent negotiations work. The idea of a consent negotiation isn't to negotiate against your connection to get what you want. It's to negotiate with your connection to get the experience that will be best for both of you.

Juan and Cho want to have sex, but Cho has had problems with consent as a process, getting so caught up she forgets to check in with her connection. She and Juan discuss this and decide to try consent as a negotiation.

They talk about what they want to do when they have sex.

Juan doesn't want dirty talk. Cho is okay with that.

Cho needs lots of foreplay because she doesn't get much from penetration. Juan is okay with that.

Juan offers to skip penetration entirely if Cho is willing to go down on him.

Cho thinks about it a bit and says she doesn't have a preference, so whichever Juan prefers. Juan prefers penetration.

It is this back and forth that makes it a negotiation, instead of each person simply setting their boundaries.

You don't need to pick just one approach to consent. You can mix and match. You can use consent-as-process for your relationship and consent-as-negotiation for kink scenes and enthusiastic consent for vanilla sex or whatever works for you.

4.2 Watch for the Landmines

No one can predict all the possible problems in any relationship. But for folks integrating polyamory and kink for the first time, there are a few common landmines to watch out for. Here are the ones I know about.

4.2.1 Your Squicks Are Yours

I hope it goes without saying by now, but so long as they respect your limits, your squicks aren't other people's problems. That means if you don't want to hear talk about something that squicks you, that's fine, you can ask for that. If you don't want your partner(s) to do something that squicks you, you need to get over that or get out of the relationship. YKINMK *and that's okay.*

The thing is, a lot of common kinks squick vanilla people. And sometimes they can't be kept away from you without doing damage to your relationship. If one of your partners is a masochist, *they are going to be sore the next day*. Possibly for the next several days. Your choice is to avoid seeing them during that period or learn to live with it. Similarly if one of your partners is in chastity. Or wears a collar. Bondage leaves pressure marks that sometimes take a while to fade. Sometimes it will leave bruises.

If you are getting into kink, or one of your partners is kinky, you need to watch for squicks and how you react to them. If you've been in polyamory a while, coping with negative emotions shouldn't be new to you. Lean in. Communicate, be honest with your partners *and with yourself*.

Obviously, this won't always apply. Sometimes the stuff that squicks you can stay behind closed doors. But we all know the deal with that, right?

If kink is something your partner can pick up or put down as they choose, then not bringing the kink on your dates isn't a problem. But if their kink is part of who they are and inherent to how they do sex and/or relationships, then you aren't asking them to keep it behind closed doors. You are asking them to keep it in the closet. Not cool. At all.

Your squicks are yours. Like your jealousy and your insecurities. Ask your partners for help dealing with them, lay boundaries as you need. But at the end of the day, you are the one who needs to deal with them.

4.2.2 The 'Me' Versus the 'We'

Something that is at the core of polyamory, but not often talked about, is separating the 'me' from the 'we.' US culture, and Anglo culture in general (can't speak for the rest of the world), treats two people in a relationship as a unit. Everything from language to social customs enforces this idea that 'two become one.'

That attitude won't work long in polyamory. You need to be able to separate yourself from your partner and both act as individuals.[11]

But that's polyamory. In The Scene, keeping a strong 'we' is

11 Note: this 'two become one' thing is different from pair bonding. Pair bonding is an emotional connection that is near universal in human experience. There are strong pair bonds in polyamory, including some folks who consider themselves part of a couple. What can't work, in the long term, is people giving up their individuality and being subsumed into the couple-unit.

very common. In fact, the Scene tends to retain many monogamous attitudes towards relationships. Including the idea that you are responsible for your partner's jealousy.

So if you have experience in polyamory, you likely have practice separating 'me' from 'we'—but your kinky partner might not. Worse, your kink partner may sense something is 'wrong' or 'different' without understanding why. They may feel insecure or slighted or like you aren't 'really into them' because you don't let yourself get lost in the 'we.'

But they likely won't have the experience or knowledge to put into words why it feels wrong to them.

You may be best off addressing this directly, rather than waiting for it to come up. 'Hey, I don't know what your experience has been, but I don't do the whole 'two people are everything to each other' thing. I am an individual, and you are an individual, and we connect with each other. If you are expecting us to become each others 'other halves' or otherwise become a single unit rather than individuals, this isn't going to work.'

Some may be relieved 'Oh, really? That's great. I usually feel smothered in relationships because of that kind of thing.'

Some may be confused, and you can either try to explain further or let it go for the time being.

Some may say they get it, but it turns out later that they didn't. Then it's, 'You remember what I said about still being an individual? This is what I meant. I'm sorry you were hurt/confused/etc about this. Can we talk about how we've each approached it differently and how we can deal with this kind of thing in the future?'

Some may not accept it, and you are probably incompatible.

4.2.3 Trauma Reactions

Lots of folks have dealt with traumas. And some traumas will cause problems with either polyamory or kink (or both!). Someone who has been cheated on may have a bad reaction to polyamory. Ditto someone who has seen a relationship implode because of supposedly-ethical-nonmonogamy-that-wasn't.

And someone who has been physically abused is not going to react well to impact play—or seeing the bruises from impact play.

We'll talk more about this in a bit, but as far as landmines go:

Almost everyone who has trauma will have unexpected

triggers. There is always something we thought we'd be okay with but aren't. If one or more of you have trauma in your history, be aware that trauma is a possible landmine that can catch you by surprise.

4.2.4 Assumptions, Assumptions, Assumptions

Just gonna hammer this home one more time. Assumptions, yours and your partner(s), will blow up in your face. Try to clear out as many as you can ahead of time. And when there is a blow-up in your relationship, make sure your first step is checking for unrecognized assumptions.

4.3 Managing Your Squicks

Alright, it's well and good for me to say 'your squicks are yours.' But that doesn't actually give you any useful information on how to deal with them.

I'm going to do my best, but to an extent, this is something that everyone will need to find their own way to navigate.

First, it's important to know where your squicks come from. I'm autistic and most new things squick me a bit. But once I've tried it a time or two I'm usually okay. Handling that is completely different from handling a squick from a cultural taboo or prior bad experience. (You know, I've been assuming this goes without saying, but I should say it to be safe—a trauma reaction is *not* a squick. Do not treat it like one.)

Make sure you talk with your partner(s) about what squicks you and why.

So, my take, and YMMV a lot here:

Most squicks can be dealt with by facing them. Exposure therapy works for a reason, after all. If it's a 'this is new' squick, then having someone you trust walk you through it a few times should be enough to help you find your feet.

If it's a cultural taboo thing, then better to work up to it gradually, but still, face it. If seeing your partner's bruises freaks you out, don't ask them to hide their bruises. Instead, look at them. Ask your partner how they feel about their bruises. Lean on that compersion thing and see how happy your partner is, how proud or giddy their bruises make them. It won't be quick or easy, but if you work at it, you can get more comfortable with it.

If you've had a prior bad experience—for a completely *random* example you tried something new and someone threw up on you (Who me? No, uh-uh, nope. Why do you ask?)[12][13] Well, if it's just a bad experience that doesn't rise to the level of trauma, you may still be a bit squicked by it.

In this case, 'get back on the horse' is a cliche for a reason. If you open yourself up to new, positive experiences, in time they will outweigh and replace the older bad experience.

Now—you don't need to get comfortable with things that squick you. If no one in your polycule is doing those things, and you aren't interested in them, there's no need to put in the effort. If someone in your 'cule is doing squicky stuff, you don't need to get comfortable with it either. Maybe they do scat play—but if they don't do it when you are around, clean up afterward, and don't about it around you, you may be okay.

But if they are doing something that leaves marks, or if you are going to be attending play parties and dungeons together where they'll be playing with other people, confronting your squicks is a good idea.

4.4 When Trauma Gets in the Way

Like I said before, a trauma reaction is completely different from a squick and shouldn't be dealt with in the same way.

A big one for trauma reaction is going to be bruises/impact play, so to keep things simple that's what we'll talk about here. But anything can cause a trauma reaction in the wrong circumstances.

4.4.1 The Necessary Caveats

First off, to steal a line from the amazing Xan West, "Survivors in a relationship trigger each other... You getting triggered by [them] is not [their] fault... Or [their] responsibility."[13] This is true for the situation Xan was writing about—two people who are both survivors. But it is also true when just one person is a survivor. Getting triggered *happens* in a relationship.

You should never blame your partner for triggering you, try to make them feel guilty, or make dealing with your trauma their responsibility. You need to be working on your own healing, setting up a support network, identifying your needs, etc.

---

12 Trying to deep throat someone with a really sensitive gag reflex is rather contraindicated...

13 Xan West, *Nine of Swords Reversed*, Chapter 4

That doesn't give your partner an excuse to be an asshole.

If they trigger you intentionally, refuse to help (within their limits and abilities) when you are triggered, or refuse to make accommodations and adjustments to help you avoid being triggered, you should 'Nope' yourself out of there. That is not a healthy relationship.

4.4.2 The Main Point

Hopefully, the above wasn't needed. Regardless, we can move on.

Here, we're assuming a generally healthy relationship, you both try to help and support each other. But *shit happens*. A person is triggered by impact play and/or bruises and a person who does impact play are trying to make their relationship work.

We are not going to discuss asking the kinky partner to give up impact play. While them stopping impact play is an option, it is not something you get to ask for. It is for them to offer, or not. Some folks need the impact play, for various reasons. If they ask *you* if giving up their impact play would help, answer honestly. But unless they have told you it's okay to ask them to stop kinky stuff that bothers you, don't ask.

However, there are other things you can ask them.

1. Keep it elsewhere: ask them to keep the stuff that triggers you elsewhere, at play parties or when visiting other partners.

2. Ask them to keep it out of sight: many kinky folks need to make sure no marks will show because of work or privacy issues. You can ask for the same. Understand that if you do want to do out-of-sight/out-of-mind, you need to accept that their clothes will be staying *on* until any bruises have time to fade.

3. Ask for a warning: asking them to let you know if they will be doing impact play or have bruises ahead of time. This gives you a chance to prepare for it.

4. Make a plan: how will you both handle it when you are triggered? What 'aftercare' will you need to help you recover?

5. Follow the advice for squicks: I went a bit too far saying you shouldn't treat trauma like a squick. The truth is that *sometimes* you can gradually expose yourself to something triggering and work past the trauma. In psychology, this is called 'exposure therapy.' But it's something you need to be ready for, have a good support system in place, and move at your own pace. You know the 'you shouldn't ask' above? Well for this, *they* shouldn't ask. This is for you to try when you are ready.

4.4.3 Your Partner Can't Completely Protect You

Look, this is real life. Shit happens. A bruise is going to peak out of someone's collar. Your partner's friend will bring up the flogging demonstration at the last play party. Hell, you may hit a bruise when you and your partner are cuddling on the couch.

Again, don't blame your partner if this happens. And have a plan for how to handle it. (A care box similar to what some folks keep for aftercare can be a great tool for this.)

4.4.4 If Your Partner Drops

As I mentioned elsewhere, sometimes people drop a day or two *after* the scene is over. If your partner drops when they are with you, and the drop is caused by your trigger, that can cause some issues. If you are okay with them talking about your trigger, then you can give them support as usual, whatever your usual is. If not, then you may need to modify the care you give or not give care at all. In that case, make sure they have access to the aftercare box/supplies. If they need someone to talk with, try to get a friend on the phone they can talk stuff out with.

4.4.5 Wrapping Up (Beyond Bruises)

Okay, like I said, we focused on impact play here because it is a common issue. I also picked it because it *does* leave marks. It's easier to keep scat play private. Ditto rape play. Regardless of what your trigger is, this will hopefully give you and your kinky partner(s) a starting place for handling it.

4.5 Aftercare/Drops

Oh, hey, we should talk about this, yeah?

Sometimes you can end up dealing with your partners' drops, even if you weren't involved in the kink play. That's because of the time delay in some folk's drop.

Now, if your partner was playing with a good play partner, that play partner may try to follow up themselves. Especially after an intense scene. So there may be a phone call a day or two after the scene to check in and make sure your partner is doing okay. Even if you usually have a policy of not taking phone calls/talking with OSOs while together, please give this one a pass. Your partner's OSO is being responsible and making sure your partner is okay. This should be appreciated, not attacked.

If their calling really is an issue, make it a policy *beforehand* that you will help your partner through any delayed drops.

Hopefully, your partner can tell you ahead of time if they tend to experience delayed drops. In that case (if you don't live together) you can choose to postpone or cancel your get together if you don't want to deal with the drop. And you shouldn't need to if you don't want to. But if you live together or if they aren't able to warn you (because shit happens) you may end up dealing with a drop.

While a drop immediately after a scene is partly physical (dehydration, low blood sugar, etc) a drop later is often purely emotional. (Unless someone didn't hydrate/rest/eat after the scene.) The body has had time to recover, now the brain reacts.

Everyone's needs when they drop are different. But for delayed drops, the big thing is usually to give support and reassurance. Warm blankets and favorite snack foods are also good. Weepiness, irritability, attacks of self-doubt, and generally being in a 'funk' are common. You don't need to do anything special. In fact, you don't need to do anything. You can leave your partner to deal with their drop themself—that's what they'd do if you weren't there and most folks are fine doing so.

But if you can help, that will often make the drop pass faster. Hold them, talk to them, share cute puppy memes. Generally, just be there for them and be an anchor they can hold to until their emotions run their course.

5 Time For a Closer Look at Power Exchange

We covered the basics of power exchange already. Now let's dig into the details. From here on, I'm using the terms d-type and s-type unless I'm referring to a specific type of power exchange relationship.

5.1 The C Word

We know that communication is important in both kink and polyamory, but it has some extra importance—and challenges—in power exchange. And the more power an s-type gives to the d-type, the more important communication becomes.

As the one making decisions, the d-type needs information to make good decisions. They can only get that information if the s-type communicates with them. However, the manner of power exchange often restricts the s-types ability to communicate. Most d-types set rules against things like refusing orders and arguing. Speech restrictions, like not speaking without permission, and use of gags aren't exactly uncommon.

To make sure that the power exchange and communication can continue, d-types often make certain that their s-type(s) has ways to express themself. Daily journaling is a common requirement for 24/7 s-types. Some d-types make a rule, or some s-types specify a limit, that allows for a 'time out' in the power exchange. They can talk about issues as equals, with the s-type returning power to d-type when they are done.

Often, power exchange is temporary, for instance, a single scene. Most of the communication takes place before the scene and after. That's the point of negotiation and some kinds of aftercare. But safewords and regular check-ins during the scene makes sure that everything is okay.

5.2 Relationship Structures

Like we covered earlier, there are four main kinds of power exchange relationships. Dominant/submissive, Master/slave, Owner/pet, and Adult/little.

Some specific types of power exchange have their own well-known names. For instance, Lady/knight is a specific type of D/s relationship. It is popular among F/m pairings who prefer a gentle and worshipful approach to D/s. Owner/puppy and Owner/pony are both popular forms of Owner/pet often referred to as 'pup play' and 'pony play.' 'Kitten play' isn't as popular (yet) but that may be changing.

D/s is in some ways the base form of power exchange. In D/s, someone gives power and someone receives power. If power exchange happens in a relationship, it can be called D/s.

M/s usually refers to 24/7 TPE relationships and may involve consensual non-consent. Not everyone who has a 24/7 TPE relationship will use M/s terminology, but you will rarely see M/s terminology used for a non-24/7 TPE relationship.

Folks debate endlessly in kinky forums and chat rooms about the difference between a submissive and a slave. It's very much a blurred line and not everyone considers it a meaningful distinction.

In pet play, the s-type takes on the role of a pet, usually a specific type of animal. You might say that pets are the furries of the kink world, people who identify with an animal. Their role as a pet allows them to live as that animal (more or less, for varying periods of time). Other people who do pet play don't see themselves as being that animal but enjoy losing themselves in the animal persona.

One of the appeals of giving up power is the freedom of not needing to worry and letting the d-type make decisions. A pet gives up a greater measure of power, often acting the animal in all ways, including not speaking and having all their physical needs cared for. This gives a greater measure of freedom to relax.

Age play or adult/little relationships tend to be the hardest for vanilla folks to understand. I wrote this for a Quora answer and it made sense to folks, so (with my known distaste for reinventing the wheel), I'll include it here:

> Some people like to take care of others. They often
> need to watch themselves in relationships because
> they can easily end up in one of two problems: being
> taken advantage of, or pissing their self-sufficient
> partner off.

> Some people like to be taken care of. Similarly, they
> can end up in problematic relationships, either by
> going with someone who is abusive in the guise of
> taking care of them, or by being too needy for their
> partners.

> Many people, regardless of their approach to
> relationships, have a very strong 'inner child,' Most of
> them are perfectly capable of 'adulting' but want to
> be able to express their child-self.

> With this, just general people stuff, no mention of
> kink, we can see how an Adult/little relationship
> might develop. Someone who likes to take care of
> people and wants a healthy relationship meets
> someone who likes being taken care of and also
> wants a healthy relationship. If the person who likes
> being taken care of also has a strong inner child, you
> have all the ingredients for an Adult/little
> relationship.

In an Adult/little relationship a person with a strong inner child gives power to someone they trust (often, but not always, a relationship partner). They can let that inner child out for a while and know that they have someone to take care of them while they take a break from adulting.

'Little' is a catch-all term. A little's 'inner child' can range from baby (diapers and all in some cases) up to teenager.

The adult in an Adult/little relationship will often use a parent title such as Mommy or Daddy, but other titles aren't unheard of.

Both Adult/little and pet play relationships can sometimes overlap with sexual role play. For instance, a sexual Teacher/student role play where the teacher has control is similar to Adult/little relationships. However, people who engage in such role-play will rarely identify as Adult/little. Role play is role play, being little is usually part of a person's identity. And many folks who do identify as Adult/little are primarily in their power exchange roles outside the bedroom. Some don't take the roles in the bedroom at all—though many do.

The types of power exchange don't need to be separated. For instance, my pet and I have a D/s relationship. I call them pet because we both prefer the implication of affection and emotional bonds in having a pet. But in our regular dynamic, I am not her owner, I am her dom and my title is Miss. Sometimes, however, we will swap roles for a bit and she will let her pup-side out to play. Then I will be her Owner for the period of a scene while we enjoy something different. I have known folks who mixed A/l and D/s into a unique 24/7 relationship style where the s-type could be both little and submissive at all times. Like polyamory, there are a million and one ways to do a power exchange.

Terms for power exchange relationships:

24/7: a relationship where the power exchange is constant until and unless someone stops it.

Bedroom-only: a relationship where the power exchange is part of sex and doesn't happen outside of sex/sexual interactions

Collared/Collaring: For many power exchange relationships, collaring is analogous to getting married. Many kinky folks have included a collaring ceremony in their wedding. Being collared or having a collaring ceremony is different from wearing a collar. Any s-type can and may wear a collar, whether for a specific scene, event, or because the d-type likes the way it looks. A collaring ceremony is a significant moment in the relationship.

Collaring has other meanings in other subcultures, in particular, it is a more casual thing in the furry community. Also, some folks in BDSM will do 'training collars' or other temporary collarings.

High protocol: a power exchange with a lot of rules. Specifically many rules about how the s-types acts around and addresses the d-type, and vice-versa.

Some events are called 'high protocol.' At a high protocol play party where s-types are expected to not look at any d-type (keep their eyes down)s and not speak unless invited. Other rules may apply depending on the event and venue. A switch will need to pick one role for the event and stay in that role.

Low protocol: a relationship with little or no rules about how the s-type can act around or address the d-type.

A low protocol event has no rules for s-types beyond those set by their d-types.

Contrary to what you see in BDSM novels, most events and clubs are low protocol. Folks in the Scene recognize that not everyone is into power exchange.

Total power exchange: a relationship where the d-type has complete control of the s-type, including every aspect of their life. Expected in relationships identified as M/s.

Training: a temporary power exchange to teach an s-type the behavior and protocol expected by a d-type. Since every d-type has a different idea of what they want, training is more talked about than done. Most often seen in communities that all use the same protocols, such as Gorean.

Common Titles:

Dominant: d-type in a D/s relationship

Submissive: s-type in a D/s relationship

Dom/Domme: short for dominant, dom can be either masculine or gender-neutral, domme is feminine. No, it is not pronounced 'dom-ay.' Never, absolutely forbidden by my power as Self Appointed Arbiter of All Things Kink! (Okay, yes, some people pronounce it 'dom-ay.' Hurts my ears every time.)

Sub: short for submissive

Femdom/Femsub: a woman who is dominant/submissive

Maledom/Malesub: a man who is dominant/submissive

Enbydom/Enbysub: a nonbinary person who is dominant/submissive. (Not common. As far as I know, I made these up, but I know several other nonbinary folks in power exchange and we need something to call ourselves!)

Dominatrix: Usually professional femdom, may or may not be into power exchange when off the clock. Sometimes another word for femdom.

Master/Mistress: d-type in an M/s relationship or title of respect an s-type uses for their d-type. Outside of a relationship, can be a community title of respect for a d-type who has been around a while and earned general recognition.

Slave: s-type in an M/s relationship

Owner: d-type in an O/p relationship

Pet: s-type in an O/p relationship

Adult: d-type in an A/l relationship

Little: s-type in an A/l relationship

A note on pony play: other types of power exchange relationships can be done in your regular clothes, or no clothes, with fetish gear being optional. For pony play, a certain amount of (often expensive) gear is generally expected and sometimes required. You can't 'drive' or 'ride' your pony without reins, after all. This can make pony play off-putting to new folks. Especially when you see the rigs the folks who've been in it for years have amassed. That said, many pony play forums are welcoming to new ponies, with or without gear.

I want to note that the terms and titles used here are for clarity only. A pet can call their owner 'Master.' Sometimes a dom will call their sub 'pet.' Littles don't call their adult 'Adult,' they'll use 'Mommy' or 'Daddy' most often, and sometimes other titles as they see fit. So if someone talks about having a 'master,' don't assume they are a slave (and vice-versa). Each relationship will have its own titles which may have nothing to do with that relationship type is discussed in the Scene.

5.3 Talking About Dominants

Folks new to BDSM tend to be confused by the many words for 'dominant.' After all, there's only one term for 'submissive' why are there a half dozen terms for dominant?

Largely it's because of how many people have assumed that dominant=man. Because of the notoriety of the gay leather scene, few are surprised by a male sub. Many still insist that a dominant woman 'hasn't met the right man yet. Women who were dominant started coming up with their own variations on 'dominant' and 'dom' to make it clear that yes, they were women, and dominant.

Several years ago, some of us in a Fetlife forum for women who love submissive men tried to get 'subbe' going as meaning a male sub. It didn't go anywhere, but it did draw attention to the ridiculousness of the gendered assumption many people have about dominants. (Yes, misogyny seems to be the same everywhere.)

5.4 The Appeal of Power Exchange

We've looked at what power exchange is, but what's the appeal? Why do people want to do it?

Control is generally seen as the main appeal of power exchange relationships. It's right there in the definitions: doms like to control, subs like to be controlled.

Most non-kinky people assume that 'like' in this case means 'are sexually aroused by.' For many people, there is some truth to that. However, it isn't sexual for everyone and folks for whom it is sexual for often like it for other reasons as well. Each person comes to power exchange with a different idea of what they want.

Aside from control, the two aspects of power exchange that appeal to many people are obedience and service.

Obedience is relatively straight forward. D-types are obeyed, s-types obey. For many s-types, obedience is relaxing, even freeing in a way. When you obey you don't need to figure things out, worry if you are doing the right thing, stress over all the other stuff you 'should' be doing right then. You can forget everything, knowing that your d-type is responsible for all that stuff, and focus on doing the job you were told to do. For d-types, honestly, it's pretty much a straight-up power trip. But better than a vanilla power trip because of a fun-house mirror effect. Your s-type likes you having power, so you get feels over having the power and compersion-type happy over making your s-type feel good with the power. That makes you enjoy the power more because you used the power in a way that made this person you care for feel good. And round and round it goes. (This plays out other ways in degradation and humiliation play, but the general pattern is the same.)

Service is a whole other 'ball of wax.' The general assumption is that the s-type serves and the d-type is served. But like all assumptions, that one can bite you on the ass.

First, because that's not the way it works, at all, in many A/l and O/p dynamics. In those dynamics, the d-type is 'serving' the s-type. The d-type takes care of their needs, makes sure they have food, cuddles, boundaries, and whatever else is part of their dynamic.

Second, because (as I and some other folks are fond of saying) "I'm the dom, so we're doing it my way." If I want to serve my pet breakfast in bed, tuck them in at night, and spend an hour shaving them, then that's what will happen. Some d-types, even those who go by 'dom' or 'master' like taking care of their s-types. And 'taking care of' often looks exactly the same as service, the only difference being who is making the decisions.

The vast majority of power exchange relationships I am familiar with have a service dynamic, but who serves who varies. For many folks, it will vary within the dynamic. Sometimes I serve/take care of my pet, sometimes they serve/take care of me. In either case, I'm still the dom, because I'm the one saying 'okay, we're doing this today.'

This is also the appeal of power exchange that will be most

familiar to vanilla folks. Taking pleasure in control and obedience isn't something many vanilla folks are used to (or comfortable with). Taking pleasure in taking care of someone you love is known and appreciated in vanilla relationships.

5.5 Relationship Controls

For many polyamorists, the most challenging part of 24/7 power exchange to adjust to is that a d-type gets to approve their s-type's other relationships. In some cases, people need to ask a d-type's permission before approaching the s-type (on fetlife or at a play party).

This is similar enough to a veto arrangement that it gets many polyam folk's backs up. And I understand that. I don't try to control my pet's other relationships, the idea is borderline squick for me. But YKINMK.

Having said that, there are fundamental differences between a veto and relationship controls in power exchange.

In polyamory, a veto arrangement is framed as protecting the original couple and/or a way to manage jealousy. Vetoes are notorious for the way they deny a new partner agency in their relationships and generally treat them as 'second class citizens.'

Relationship controls in power exchange have none of that framing.[14]

Relationship controls are the d-type taking their responsibility seriously. Remember that in a power exchange relationship, the d-type is responsible for ensuring the s-type's wellbeing. Some folks are comfortable with the d-type saying, 'I trust you to vet your own partners, just tell me if there is a problem or you need my help. 'But some might prefer for the d-type to say, 'I know you can vet your own partners, but it's my responsibility to take care of you. So I'll be vetting them too.'

I personally am uncomfortable with that level of control in a power exchange relationship. I won't interfere with my pet's friends, relationships, or family. I have an advisory role in their path towards a full-time career, but that's no more than many a nesting partner has. A nesting partner's career impacts your life together.

But that's me.

---

14 That doesn't mean jealousy or 'protecting' a relationship is never part of the reason some d-types insist on relationship controls. Again, there are assholes and abusers in every community. But folks who do that are not the norm and not following what folks in the Scene consider 'best practices.'

If you prefer not to get involved with someone whose d-type needs to approve their new partners, that's okay. You can have that boundary. It's a boundary that many kinky people share, actually.

But some folks have different boundaries. If you meet kinky folks with relationship controls, don't get on their case about vetoes. Understand they are coming from a different place than the vetoes you are familiar with. Respect the boundaries they have for their relationship.

5.6 NonMonogamy And Power Exchange

We talked a bit earlier about how common nonmonogamy is in the Scene. In fact, it's common enough that I've heard more than one s-type vent about how frustrating it is trying to find a monogamous d-type in the Scene. My anecdotal experience is that monogamous relationships still outnumber nonmonogamous relationships. But any given time more non-mono people (d- or s-type) are open to a new relationship than mono folks. After all, a monogamous person with one relationship is unavailable for new relationships. A non-mono person with one relationship is usually still available for new relationships.

When talking about nonmonogamous power exchange, there is one thing you have to remember. *Kinky folks use a different definition of hierarchy than polyam folks do.*

In polyamory 'hierarchy' means one *relationship* having power or higher priority over another relationship. There are many ethical issues with this, they have been thoroughly explored elsewhere.

In kink, hierarchy refers to the hierarchy created by *power exchange*. One or more people have given power to one or more other people. This hierarchy exists only because all the individuals involved have decided that this is what they want. It is not a hierarchy of one relationship being 'more important' or having 'higher priority' than another relationship.

The knee jerk rejection many polyam folks have to hierarchy is going to be offputting and excluding to kinky folks. They won't understand where it is coming from and here is at a condemnation of power exchange. And polyam folks who don't understand kink hierarchy *have* taken issue with power exchange relationships. Often talking out their asses in the process. If you get that knee jerk, sit on it. Again, YKINK. Take the time to learn from the folks doing power exchange how their hierarchy works. I expect you'll find it's nothing like what you think.

Having said that, let's take a longer look at some of the more common types of nonmonogamous power exchange.

5.6.1 Kinky/'Nilla Relationships

For polyam folks who aren't kinky, this is the most common relationship structure. Kinky/'nilla is the kinky equivalent of a mono/poly relationship and has some of the same challenges.

Most polyam folks know that you can't be everything for your partner. Society teaches us that two people should be able to be everything for each other and not being able to do so is a sign of failure. Getting past this is a challenge for folks new to nonmonogamy. If you are still struggling with that, I'm afraid this may be another learning opportunity for you.

Kinky/'nilla relationships are common in polyamory and other forms of nonmonogamy. In nonmonogamy, a kinky person doesn't need to screen their partners for compatible kinks. Many kink folks, and especially power exchange folks, make the first filter of their dating life 'are they a compatible (d-type/s-type)?' This excludes a whole lot of people who might otherwise be compatible.

For people who don't need kink in every relationship, a nonmonogamous relationship opens up the dating pool. We will enjoy non-kinky stuff with our non-kinky partners and kinky stuff with our kinky partners.

The big challenge for most kinky/'nilla relationships is acceptance. This is mainly an issue if you don't understand the appeal of your partner's kinks or, worse, your partner's kinks squick you.

The exception to this will be 24/7 power exchange.

In 24/7 power exchange relationships, the d-type controls the s-types actions even when the d-type isn't there. If your partner is a d-type they will need to be aware of their s-type partner's needs. The greater the control they exert, the more they need to be available and alert to things that will affect their s-type partner.

If your partner is the s-type in a 24/7 power exchange, the d-type partner will be exerting control during your time together. Now, this may not impact your time at all. You likely won't notice. But it can impact things. At the low end, this impact can be things like 'my dom requires me to check in at 8 every night.' Intense power exchange might include rules about what kind of sex they can have, when they get up in the morning, and what they eat.

Yes, there are relationships like this. Relationships that work. Relationships where everyone is on board and supporting the dynamics that make the relationship work.

Which is not to say it's easy. Just that it happens.

Of course, most dynamics don't have that level of control. Most dynamics are only in effect when the d- and s-type are together and/or during a scene.

Unfortunately, many people transition from a vanilla monogamous relationship to a mono/poly & kinky/'nilla relationship. This often happens if someone finds they can't manage without their kink and their partner can't fill that role for them. There are worse ways to enter nonmonogamy. But going from vanilla monogamous to mono/poly & kinky/'nilla at the same time is definitely a challenge.

5.6.2 Double D/Double s

It isn't uncommon for two d-types or two s-types to end up in a committed relationship. Hopefully, they were both aware of their kink orientation and entered the relationship knowing they were incompatible in kink. However, folks often realize they are kinky only after being in a committed relationship for a while. And then discover their kinks aren't compatible.

The same issue can come up with two switches or a switch with a d- or s-type. A switch with someone who isn't a switch will only get to express one side of their power exchange kink. That works for some people, but others feel a need for both. When two switches are in a relationship, well, keep in mind that there are several ways of being a d- or s-type. A switch who is a Dom and a pet may end up in a relationship with a switch who is an Adult and a sub. They can do straight D/s together, but the Adult/pet combo may not work well.

For kinky folks who were nonmonogamous before they explored kink, this isn't a problem. For many monogamous kinky folks, this situation can push them to explore nonmonogamy.

It's common for an s-type couple to look for a d-type together. Similarly, a d-type couple may look for an s-type together.

In polyamory, a couple seeking 'a third for both of them' sets off all kinds of flags. With good reason, given the history of Unicorn Hunters in the community.

The history of couples looking together in the kink scene is different. Possibly because of the assumptions inherent in being a d- or s-type. An s-type couple looking together is expecting the d-type they find to have power over them in some way. This acts as a balancing factor to couple privilege. For d-type couples, the community-emphasis on negotiation and limits usually prevents UH-style trampling of a new s-type partner's needs.

Unfortunately, none of this stops predatory couples, it only mitigates thoughtless couples. The Scene has its share of predatory couples, both d-types and s-types. And they can do a shit ton of damage to anyone they get their hands on.

It's much rarer for a couple of switches to go looking together for a new partner. If only because one person is unlikely to be compatible with them both—even less likely than usual for couples 'seeking a third.' A couple of switches will be more likely to look for other people to create a staircase or household set up.

5.6.3 One D-type, Many S-types

It is common for a d-type to have multiple s-types serving them/in their care. Two or more d-types with a single s-type happens, but it's rarer.

Sometimes in these setups, one s-type will have a special position, referred to as the 'alpha sub.' The specifics of the alpha's role will vary. In general, they will have some power over other s-types and have extra responsibilities to the d-type.

Some of these groups call themselves, 'harems,' but it isn't a universal term. Often these groups refer to themselves as a family. If the relationships are O/p focused, stable, kennel, or other animal-based terms might be used.

Harem is, in fact, a very problematic term. It was historically used to exotify and 'other' non-European cultures, which is bad enough. Worse, how the word 'harem' is used in English has nothing to do with what a historical harem was. A 'harem' was simply the area of a palace reserved for the women who lived there. Most of those women were *not* wives or concubines of the ruler.

5.6.4 Staircases

Staircases are a chain of relationships that don't directly interact (in a kinky sense). Staircases can take a parallel approach, a kitchen table approach, or anything in between, but there are clear boundaries in the D/s aspects. It's called a staircase because the kink relationships often 'descend' like stairs—A is dom to B who is dom to C who is dom D. But it doesn't need to be linear. The main point is that A is dom to *B*. Not to C or D. And C subs to B, but not to A.

Staircases are common for switches and can take any (or even several) D/s forms.

In my family, we had a small staircase. I (and Michon) are doms and owners to Michael. Michael was dom to Ericka. Michon and I had *no* kinky relationship with Ericka. We could not give her orders, did not expect service from her, etc. We interacted with her as we would with anyone else we knew. Not as doms and a sub.

This is different from a 'harem' with an alpha sub. In a 'harem,' Michael would have been *appointed* by the d-type. Instead, her being dom to Ericka is something she and Ericka agreed on.

This is also different from a household (coming up next) where dominance and submission are transitive.

5.6.5 Households

So let's look at households.

A D/s household involves multiple people in power exchange and can include multiple d-types, switches, and s-types. Unlike a staircase, there is *one* power exchange agreement that they all take part in. There will be a set of house rules that apply to everyone. And a hierarchy of power exchange within the household. The head of the household has power over everyone below them. Someone in the middle gives power to those above them and has power over those below them. The person at the bottom gives power to everyone above them.

Each household will have their own way of establishing hierarchy. I have never been privileged to see or interact with a house for an extended period. Those I have learned a bit of didn't share their specific rules and approaches publicly. However, the hierarchy wasn't set by the head of the house assigning a ranking to each member. My impression is that most households determine ranking through a combination of negotiation and what everyone is comfortable with. My own family is taking a similar approach as we transition to more of a household set up.

5.6.6 Gor

I nearly forgot to include Gor in here, and I kind of wish I didn't remember. But it's a thing that you might run into.

Gor is an approach to kink and BDSM based on the misogynistic fantasy books by John Norman. The books are set on a counter-Earth called Gor. Most of the women depicted in the Gor books are slaves of the men and/or the city they live in. All Gorean relationships are Master/slave and most of them are M/f.

The Gorean subculture in kink draws heavily on these books. Thankfully, most Goreans recognize the books as fiction and not a how-to guide. The vast majority of Gorean relationships are M/f, a few are F/m or same-sex relationships. The amount of misogyny you will run into varies with the Gorean group. Some are extremely misogynist, pushing the idea that slavery comes naturally to women and mastery naturally to men. Other groups take the practices of Gor and try to leave behind much of the misogynistic philosophy.

Gor is fairly unique in the Scene for having a shared ritualized aspect. Many power exchange relationships include a degree of ritual, but each relationship is making up those rituals as they go along. Many folks who want ritual in their power exchange without wanting to create it from the whole cloth. Gorean relationships are one of the only places to find that. For instance, Gor has standardized slave positions for different situations and purposes. In the Scene, two different non-Gor masters who ask a slave to 'present'[15] often expect different things. But Gor has a specific position for that which all Gorean masters will use. Gor also has its own jargon drawn from the Gor books. For instance, a female slave is called a kajira and a male slave is called a kajirus.

However, the misogyny runs fairly deep in Gor. At this point, it's a bit chicken-and-egg. People who aren't comfortable with misogyny avoid Gor, so most Goreans are misogynist, causing people who aren't comfortable with misogyny to avoid Gor...

Polyamory culture and ethics were grown out of and shaped by feminism. Gorean relationships would probably be the most difficult type of D/s to integrate into a polyamorous relationship.

In terms of nonmonogamy, Gor relationships are arguably a subset of 'One D-type, many s-type.' But I figured given the.... peculiarities of Gorean relationships they should have a separate heading.

5.7 Twue D/s

15 Position themselves in a way that displays their body for inspection.

Sadly, just like everywhere, some kinksters try to insist that only some people are 'true' Doms and subs or 'truly' doing power exchange.

We're going to review a few of the common versions of twueness so you know what to look out for and avoid.

Twueness based on activity:

For some reason, certain activities got tagged as 'dominant' and some activities got tagged as 'submissive.' For instance, it's common to hear someone say that giving oral is a submissive thing and real d-type doesn't do it.

Nope. If I want to go down on my pet I will. Benefits of being the dom—I get what I want. (Within all stated limits and boundaries, of course.)

Twueness based on gender:

There is definitely a strain of folks in the Scene who think that any woman who is a dom 'just hasn't found the right man yet.'

And some folks buy into the idea that all women are superior to all men. Therefore all men should submit to all women—whether the women in question wants them to or not.

No. Anyone can fill any role, regardless of gender (or lack thereof).

Twueness based on appearance:

I've seen femdoms get this more than maledoms (for better or worse there is no stereotypical enbydom look yet) but maledoms can get it too. If you don't dress the right way, have the right look, etc, in some people's eyes, you aren't a real dom. S-types, in my experience, get less of this bullshit over the way they dress, but larger s-types and/or well-muscled s-types can get shit. Many folks think that a large physique means someone should be a d-type and there is something wrong with them for wanting to submit.

Hell no. I can dom while tied up in a chest harness and wearing a collar if I want to. And Mr. Universe can sub (or be a little, pony, or slave) if he wants to.

Twueness based on equipment:

This is a particular problem in pony play, though it's definitely heard in other power exchange relationships. To some people, if you don't have the 'right' equipment you aren't a twue. In pony play, the expectation is primarily on the pony, who is pushed to have lots of tack and costume. It's also somewhat on the Owner, though from what I've heard, less so. In D/s, the dom is expected to have a huge toy chest, fancy bondage furniture, and a dungeon with a rack in the basement of their third-floor apartment. Otherwise, they aren't a 'twue' dom. (There's a reason doms are almost always rich in BDSM romances, and it's NOT just because billionaires are sexy.)

Reality: while some kinks need toys, power exchange of any variety can be done with nothing but your naked bodies. That doesn't mean the toys and tools aren't fun and awesome. They are. But power exchange is in the heart and mind, not the toys.

Twueness based on ableism:

You can't be a dom in a wheelchair, how can you beat your sub?! (Ignoring the fact that not all D/s relationships involve pain play.) I've heard similar claims for various mental illnesses, physical problems, etc,. This is commonly phrased as 'If you can't hold a job, maintain your house and have control of your life, you can't be a dom. If you can't control yourself why should anyone trust you to control them?'

Disabled and chronically ill people can and do engage in all varieties of power exchange happily and safely.

However...

Like many wrong things, there's a drop of truth here that people have built up into an ocean of lies. Unmanaged mental illness can leave you not in control of your actions. That's not safe for scening and may not be safe for 24/7 D/s. That doesn't mean people with mental illnesses can't be d-types. It means some people with undiagnosed or out of control mental illnesses should not be d-types. Sadly, undiagnosed mental illnesses are, well, undiagnosed. In my experience, most people who have been diagnosed and working to control their mental illness will be okay. And working to control does not *just* mean 'on medication.' Not everyone with mental illness needs medication. And medication on its own is rarely enough. Obviously, this is not universal, there are exceptions. Be honest with yourself about your ability to play safely (whether or not you have a diagnosis) before entering a power exchange.

Twueness based on 24/7

Some people in 24/7 power exchange insist that if it isn't 24/7 it isn't real power exchange. A common thing I've heard from these folks is that if you aren't willing to do stuff you don't want to do, you aren't submitting. This attitude misunderstands what happens in bedroom-only PE relationships. The s-type does submit, will things they don't desire to please their d-type, does not dictate what the scene is or what they want to happen in it.

That the submission is temporary doesn't make it any less real.

That isn't to say that there aren't people who like to play at being submissive rather than actually submit. This is a thing and the source of many delightful role-playing scenes. And yes, some people confuse that with submission. But that isn't a reason to dismiss or deny the true submission (and dominance) of many folks who only have PE in the bedroom.

5.8 D/s as a Job

Like the title says, for some folks D/s is a job. Best known for this are 'dominatrixes' and 'pro-dommes.' Women who get paid to act as a dominant in a scene or scenes. Pro-dommes may or may not include sexual activities among their services, so don't assume, ask. A few pro-dommes will take jobs mentoring a couple/triad/quad/etc that are exploring kink and want some guidance. No one talks about female pro-subs, but many sex workers who never claim the title of sub fill that role. I've heard of male pro-doms but never known any. I expect that non-kinky sex working men are just as used to filling a submissive role as their sisters. 'He who has the gold makes the rules,' and all that.

For some professional D/s folks, it's a job. At the end of the day, they hang up their D/s hat and go back to their private vanilla lives. For others, it's a way to get paid doing what they love.

If your partner is thinking of becoming a pro or you are thinking of entering a relationship with a pro, then you both need to have a long talk about comfort zones and boundaries. Understand that this is their job and you need to respect that. If they have an established practice that includes sexual services, and you can't handle that, you need to show yourself out. If they are still thinking about going pro, you can, of course, express any reservations or boundaries. But you need to respect that this is their decision, not yours. (Unless you're already their d-type and have negotiated such control, in which case I shouldn't need to tell you this stuff.)

Sex work shaming is a thing in polyam circles.[16] Though, less of a thing than in the mainstream. Watch yourself and your community. Sex work is a job, like any other. Don't be shitty.

---

16 Pro D/s folks are split on whether those who don't offer sexual services should be called sex workers. Some are fine with it, some aren't. I'm sure there are others with other opinions that I haven't heard from folks who consider it not worth arguing over. However, many vanilla folks won't make the distinction and will spread their shaming freely.

6 Kink and Polyamory – When a Partner Is in Power Exchange

As we've seen, power exchange relationships can challenge polyamory's most basic assumptions of what makes a 'good' relationship.

Hierarchy! Rules! Controlling people!

Horrors! Abuse! Unethical! How could you!

Especially with high levels of power exchange (PE), nonmonogamous power exchange can look a lot like unicorn hunting. You've got rules for when the s-type can have sex, who they can be in relationships with, how they interact with their d-type...

Hopefully by now you understand how different the rules in PE are from unicorn hunting. If not, I'll be diving deep into that in a few minutes.

But what a lot of people miss is that *less* impactful power exchange can actually make for more drama when you mix it with polyamory. The obvious stuff is, well, *obvious*. If you start a relationship with someone in chastity, you know upfront that you have a lot of adjustments to make.

The less obvious stuff sneaks up on you. You think that you're fine with whatever your partners' are doing in their relationship, it doesn't affect you and your relationship with them. Then you get together all three of you one evening and you see partner A kneeling at the partner B's feet and deferring to them the whole time. And maybe it freaks you out a bit.

And when the impact isn't obvious, when it sneaks up on you, it can mess things up even more than when it is obvious. See:

assumptions (again).

So, let's get into this.

6.1 Power Exchange in the Bedroom

Getting the easy one out of the way. If one of your partners does bedroom-only power exchange with another partner, go back and re-read the first section on kink and polyamory. Bedroom only power exchange in a different part of your polycule is going to impact your relationship the same as any other kink. Don't stress about it, set a boundary that you want to be informed if the PE expands beyond the bedroom. You're good.

6.2 24/7 Power Exchange

As we've covered before, power exchange relationships where the rules apply all the time are generally called 24/7 relationships. However, in most 24/7 relationships, the s-type won't *actually* be following rules 24/7. For instance, Michael and I are very low protocol and low intensity in our power exchange. When I refer to her as 'pet' I am invoking the power exchange and whatever I tell her to do is an order. Each morning, I give her a list of tasks for the day. Beyond that, we don't have any rules and often hours or an entire day can go by when she isn't actively obeying me.

In spite of how minimal this is, it's still considered 24/7 because I am in control at all times. I simply don't *exercise* that control often. Both of us would prefer a more intense and protocol-based power exchange, but given life situation, this is what works for us for now. In the future, we may (hopefully will) bump things up a bit.

Most 24/7 relationships are low key. Maybe not as low key as Michael and I are, but high protocol relationships with rules governing every aspect of the s-type's day aren't that common.

Your partner being in 24/7 PE will likely have an impact on your relationship with them. How much of an impact will vary with the type of power exchange and intensity.

6.2.1 Rules vs Rules

Alright, rules have a bad reputation among polyamory advice givers, and for good reason. Rules, after all, are frequently a means to control people. And controlling people *without their consent* is abuse.

We're all on the same page with this, right? Nonconsensual

control=Abuse. Abuse=Bad. If I need to explain more than this, you need to put this book down, go read some relationship 101 and come back in a year or two.

So it can be offputting when a partner in power exchange starts talking about having rules—either rules they need to follow or rules they impose on someone else. And even *more* offputting when the inequitable nature of the rules gets rubbed in your face. After all, rules aren't always bad, when everyone agrees to them, etc etc, but one person imposing rules on another? Rules that are only applied to the s-type partner?

(Are we leaning in yet? There you go. Take a deep breath. Lean just a bit more.)

Remember that what matters here is consent. Remember that in a healthy power exchange relationship, the s-type and d-type negotiated this. They agreed on what kind of rules everyone wanted and exactly how much control the s-type wanted to give up.

Yes, if folks in vanilla relationships started talking about rules the way PE folks do, you would have every reason to be concerned.

Power exchange relationships are a different kettle of fish. The people involved consented to (and likely sought out!) a relationship with these kinds of rules.

Having said this, your boundaries still apply. You do not need to be okay with whatever rules exist in other people's power exchange relationships—especially if those rules impact your relationship with them. And, any folks who are doing healthy power exchange should understand if you say so. Say, 'I'm not comfortable with this. Can we sit down and talk about how your power exchange is impacting our relationship and maybe negotiate something that works for everyone?' Then see what happens.

6.2.2 Responsibilities Matter

I've mostly talked about how the submissive side of power exchange impacts a relationship, the rules and tasks an s-type adheres to. But power exchange relationships often require a great deal from the d-type as well. Being given control is a responsibility. Every area of life that a d-type has control in an area they are responsible for.

This can mean being home at 9 to tuck a little into bed, or reviewing a slave's daily tasks, or checking in on a sub after an intense scene. A good d-type takes their responsibility seriously.

In theory, this shouldn't impact your relationship with a d-type more than any other commitment and responsibility. For instance, it will have much less impact than a full-time job or child care! But some folks will react badly to a d-type's responsibilities limiting what they do in a relationship. 'S-type is an adult, they can do without you one weekend!' or 'Why do you always have to call them first thing in the morning?'

A d-type's responsibilities may impact your relationship with them. This impact can range from 'not at all' to 'significantly.' Again, if the impact on your relationship with them is more than you can accept, communicate!

7 More About Power Exchange

We've talked about power exchange in general terms. Now we're going to delve into details. How do power exchange relationships work? And what should you look for in healthy power exchange?

7.1 Dealing with Problems in Power Exchange Relationships

Problems happen in relationships. We all know this. Everyone has different ways of dealing with relationship problems, but communication is usually key.

Which is, of course, why it's a core concept to both polyamory and kink.

However, power exchange relationships add extra difficulty to communication. Put simply, it can be very easy for a D-type to be unaware of or ignore a problem. Especially when the relationship has rules in place that restrict an s-types ability to discuss a problem.

Even when rules don't keep an s-type from talking about a problem, it is very common for an s-type to try to 'just get over it.' For many s-types, there is a lot of self-esteem/self-worth bound up in being a *good* s-type. If they can't do what their d-type wants, if they need to say 'no' to something, if they can't figure out a problem themselves or need to interfere or inconvenience their d-type... well, many s-types will just keep quiet about it.

Remember 'Responsibilities Matter?' This is part of why it's so important. Making sure that this communication happens is a key part of d-type responsibilities. The s-type needs to feel safe bringing up problems, not feel like having problems makes them a failure as an s-type, etc.

It isn't uncommon for d-type in a relationship to have similar-but-opposite issues. 'If I was a good dom this wouldn't be a problem.' 'A real master wouldn't need help.' and so on and so forth.

Up to a point, the d-type *is* the d-type, who chose to take on responsibility in this relationship. They need to live up to that responsibility.

As such, they need to get over themselves and open up about whatever problems they are having.

But helping the d-type get past these kinds of hang-ups is a kind of service, and such falls into the s-types bailiwick.

All the above being a really complicated way of saying:

Both sides of power exchange can get caught up in the *idea* of power exchange and forget that humans need help sometimes. And both sides of power exchange have to make sure communication is happening. If they don't, problems won't get dealt with.

But... we're human. We forget sometimes.

Whether you are part of the power exchange or not, if you see this kind of thing happening, a loving clue-by-four may be just what your partner(s) need to realize that they are being foolish. Don't be afraid to lay it on them.

7.1.1 Common Problems in PE relationships

Alright, we've touched on one common problem in power exchange relationships—lack of communication because someone thinks needing help is bad. Let's take a look at some other problems that are common in power exchange and especially nonmonogamous power exchange. (For now, we're looking at problems in otherwise *healthy* power exchange.)

7.1.1.1 Conflicting Orders/Expectations

Conflicts happen—but some conflicts we set each other up for (with or without realizing it). Especially conflicts in what we ask for or expect from our partners.

1. Polyamory Version

Some guy over in the Middle East once said that a man cannot have two masters: he will either love one and hate the other or hate one and love the other. I'm happy to say that this old dude was wrong. It is very possible to have two Masters (or two Mistresses, or a Master and a Mistress, or... hell, you get the idea.) But, it does come with some challenges.

And the biggest challenge is when the two d-types aren't on the same page and give conflicting orders or set conflicting expectations.

This problem is easy to prevent—as long as you plan ahead.

NonMonogamous power exchange relationships have developed several approaches to this.

My family prefers an explicit social hierarchy in addition to our BDSM hierarchy. So one person, Michon, is the head of the family. If Michon and I give Michael conflicting orders, Michael is to follow Michon's orders and to make sure we both know about the conflict.

That's one approach, and one that has worked well for us so far. Of course, Michael and I live together and Michon is an LDR for us, so there aren't many opportunities for conflict. When we all live together in a few years, we may need to adjust things.

If following Michon's orders first starts causing problems, we might set a safeword. We usually use the stoplight system for safewords, but it's always possible to add in some more colors. So we might say that 'purple' is the safeword for conflicting orders, and then we could stop and talk about the conflict and how to resolve it.

If most conflicts are minor things (I tell Michael to stop and drink some water and Michon tells Michael to get the kids' shoes on) we might just say that Michael will follow the first order given. Then she can go back and follow the second order.

2. Monogamy version

It's easier for two d-types to contradict each other. But one d-type can manage it just fine. Sometimes a person forgets. Sometimes the way an order is phrased will cause confusion. Or a miscommunication can create an apparent conflict.

Sometimes the d-type has some self-awareness issues. They may have conflicting expectations they aren't aware of.

In some ways, this is harder to deal with than the nonmonogamous version. When there are two d-types in a relationship, folks know to expect these kinds of conflicts, and plan for them. When there is only one d-type, few people expect or plan for that one d-type to contradict themself!

When it does happen, usually the s-type will need to point out that it did happen. If they aren't able to point it out right away, they need to do their best to manage the conflict on their own until there is a chance to discuss it. In some cases 'managing the conflict' will mean safewording. For instance, if the conflict crosses their limits or causes problems they aren't able to deal with.

Sometimes it's an ongoing issue, like if a d-type who has trouble remembering things. (Maybe they have executive dysfunction because of a health issue. Maybe they are 'just' dealing with a lot of life stress and expectations that make it hard to remember everything. They could have bad short term memory. Or whatever. Doesn't matter why.) In that case, the strategies I mentioned above for conflicting orders between two d-types can help.

3. Funishment version

'Funishment' is when everyone in the relationship wants the s-type to get in trouble because getting 'punished' is fun. Fun punishment. Funishment. You get it.

Sometimes a d-type will give conflicting or impossible orders as a set-up for funishment. So if you see conflicting orders or expectations in someone else's relationship, don't assume it's a problem.

If you are concerned, you can always check in with one of them and make sure everything is okay.

7.1.1.2 Incomplete Negotiations

This one is almost inevitable in a long-running PE. You can, with reasonable surety, negotiate everything you need to for a single scene. When you are doing PE over a long time, you are going to miss some things. My first experience with this involved funishment.

I was setting a sub up for funishment with some impossible-to-achieve orders. But I forgot we hadn't talked about funishment and this sub thought (or said he thought—more on that later) that he was failing me. He felt like he was a bad sub and should stop being my sub if he couldn't follow orders.

This kind of thing is common. You can't cover everything that might come up in a relationship in a few conversations, or even a bunch of conversations. And it's worse when time makes memories fuzzy. Maybe you thought leather cuffs were covered and your partner thinks they weren't. Also, people change—you agree to some low-key bratting, but nothing too heavy. Then your s-type finds they really like being a brat and keeps upping the brat level. Or a change in another relationship means that someone has less/more time/spoons/etc and that affects the power exchange relationship.

When this happens, it goes back to communication. First, speaking up as soon as someone notices a problem, and second renegotiating to figure out how to address it.

7.1.2 Tools to Keep Communication Flowing

Polycules sometimes need to take an active effort to keep communication flowing. Similarly, power exchange relationships often need tools to help everyone communicate. I'm not going to spend too long on this. My point is to give you an idea of the range of options available, as well as some reassurance. Even when an s-type isn't allowed to question orders, a good d-type has ways they can voice problems and concerns.

1. Many d-types will have a standing order for their s-type to tell them if they are having any problems or concerns.

2. Many s-types keep journals that their d-types will review. If they don't feel comfortable bringing up a problem, they can write about it in their journal and know their d-type will see it.

3. Like some polyam folks, many folks in power exchange will have regular check-in times. A scheduled discussion for touching base, bringing up any problems and renegotiating as needed. It isn't unheard of for d-types to institute a nightly check-in of this sort. Especially with done one-on-one, the check-in isn't likely to take much time. As long as things are going well, and a nightly check or weekly in lets them catch problems early.

You'll notice most of these are geared towards helping the s-type communicate. That's because they are giving up control, which may make it harder for them to communicate. But most communication tools work well for a d-type. They can keep a journal, or text a running account of their day, or drop notes in a suggestion box, or discuss their concerns during a check-in... or lots of other stuff, if they don't feel comfortable blurting out whatever is on their mind.

7.1.2.1 Tools Need to Be Used

A d-type can do all in their power to foster communication, but that can only do so much. As Daniel commented to me, "Self-effacing self-doubt and lack of assertiveness can be a problem even when the d-type does all in their power to open up space for communication."

Too much of porn and fiction depicts s-types as either brats who need to be forced to obey, or, well, doormats. People who have completely subsumed their personality in service to their d-type. Unfortunately, some s-types take similar ideas into their relationships.

It is the s-types responsibility to *use* the tools a d-type provides them, as well as, you know, their own basic communication skills.

Related to this—the s-type has a responsibility to be aware of themself, their needs, and how they are doing. They can't communicate if they don't have the self-awareness to know what needs to be communicated. D-types aren't mind readers. They can't sit an s-type down and force them to discuss what is wrong if the d-type isn't aware there is a problem.

7.2 Stereotypes, Bias, and Other Unhealthy Tropes

One thing polyamory doesn't have too much of (yet) is internal stereotypes. People who aren't polyamorous sure have a lot of stereotypes and biases about *us*. But there is nothing in polyamorous circles about how solo polyam folks are all standoffish, or MFM triads are more stable than FMF triads, or women get into polyamory because they are man-haters... No one expects a buff man to be in a group relationship and a feminine woman to be solo poly... you get what I'm saying.

Well, there are *lots* of stereotypes and bias like that in kink.

Like the idea that a *real* masochist doesn't safeword. Or (of course), men are doms and women are subs. (I guess that makes enbies switches?) Or that a femdom will be a cruel sadist who loves grinding a man under her heel.

There's nothing wrong with folks who fit these stereotypes. Plenty of big, tough guys are doms, and good for them. But sometimes the big, tough guy is a sub. Because people!

Of course, there are also those stereotypes and biases that mainstream culture projects onto power exchange. You've probably heard a few of those yourself. We'll be taking a look at the more common stereotypes and biases so you know what you might run into, and what you might need to unlearn.

7.2.1 Internal Stereotypes and Bias

We're going to knock this one out quickly. The basic answer to all these stereotypes is that people are people, in all their glorious variety.

1. D-types are sadists

2. s-types are masochists

3. D-types are men

4. s-types are women

5. Malesubs aren't real men

6. Femdoms are cold-hearted bitches

7. Femdoms just haven't found the *right* man

8. Maledoms are big and strong

9. Malesubs are small and wimpy

10. A d-type who switches isn't a *real* d-type

11. Bedroom-only power exchange isn't *real* power exchange

12. Men are puppies, women are ponies and kitties

13. F/f power exchange doesn't exist

14. There are way more hetero malesubs than femdoms (this may be true in some local communities, but by and large, no.)

7.2.2 External Stereotypes and Bias

Unsurprisingly, the world-at-large projects a lot of assumptions on power exchange. First, because power exchange and S&M are the only kinks that most folks outside the Scene are aware of. Second, because power exchange challenges some of the modern world's basic assumptions. So we'll go into a bit more detail about these stereotypes and biases, as well as why they are wrong and what the reality is.

7.2.2.1 Power Exchange Is Abuse

We talked about the myth that kink is abusive earlier, with a focus on S&M. But there's more to abuse than physical abuse. We all know this.[17] Abuse is about stripping another person of their agency. The types of abuse are different only in the tools the abuser uses.

Power exchange is all about control, and yeah, it can look like abuse from the outside. Just like polyamory can look like cheating sometimes.

Again, consent is key. That doesn't mean power exchange relationships can't be abusive. Just like people can cheat in polyamory, abuse can happen in power exchange. We'll be looking at how you can recognize abuse in power exchange a

---

17 If you didn't when you started reading, you'd better know it now!

little later. But power exchange itself isn't abuse.

Hopefully by now, I didn't need to write all this. But, ya know, better safe.

7.2.2.2 It's a Mental Illness

There's an idea that floats around about how kinky folks in general and power exchange folks in particular must have some kind of mental illness. (We talked about the S&M version of this earlier.) Well, we have actual science to answer this question. A study done several years ago found that d-types are, on average, mentally healthier than s-types. And *both* are, on average, mentally healthier than the non-kinky control group.

> The results mostly suggest favorable psychological characteristics of BDSM practitioners compared with the control group; BDSM practitioners were less neurotic, more extraverted,[18] more open to new experiences, more conscientious, less rejection sensitive, had higher subjective well-being, yet were less agreeable. Comparing the four groups, if differences were observed, BDSM scores were generally more favorably for those with a dominant than a submissive role, with least favorable scores for controls.

From *Psychological characteristics of BDSM practitioners* by Andreas Wismeijer and Marcel Van Assen, published in the Journal of Sexual Medicine.[19]

Now, this is a single study, and *repeatability* is the core of science. That said, this study involved over a thousand people and was a follow-up to other, smaller-scale studies.

So unless actual evidence of mental illness around power exchange crops up, it's safe to lay this myth to rest.

7.2.2.3 The Limits of Power Exchange

I think many people would be surprised at how common 24/7 power exchange is. What isn't common is what many people associate with 24/7—*total* power exchange. Total power exchange, or TPE, is when the d-type has control over every aspect of the s-type's life.

Even in TPE, the s-type's limits still apply. But TPE requires

---

18 Extraverted isn't more healthy that introverted, damn it!

19 J Sex Med. 2013 Aug;10(8):1943-52. doi: 10.1111/jsm.12192. Epub 2013 May 16.

that the limits be specific. 'No rules that interfere with my family and my relationships with them,' means this relationship isn't TPE. The limit sections off a large section of the s-types life as out of the d-types control. But a TPE relationship might have a limit of 'No rules or orders that interfere with my weekly phone call with my mother.'

To put it another way, in TPE, the d-type will have control of everything not excluded by the s-type's limits. In non-TPE, the d-type will have control only of those things the s-type explicitly gives them control over. (Or that the d-type doesn't renounce control over. I've had subs who wanted to do TPE. I've always said, "That's fine, but I'm never going to control your other relationships or family stuff.")

7.2.2.4 Dominant Man=Good, Dominant Woman=Evil

Do I really need to deconstruct this one? Media, visual media especially, loves putting women villains in leather with a whip.

There has been one (1) portrayal of a woman in leather with a whip as a non-villain that most folks are aware of. Lady Heather on CSI was a huge moment for a lot of femme dominants and femdoms. But it was, of course, a one-off character, never to be repeated in other media again. I have a vague memory, from back in the last century, of a cop-comedy where the cops had to go undercover at a BDSM resort and the woman pretended to be a dom. Catwoman started as the evil villainess in leather with a whip and morphed into a beloved anti-hero. That is the sum total of my knowledge of not-evil femdoms in popular culture. Nearly 20 years looking for femdoms in media, I can name three that weren't (always) villains.

It's no surprise, of course, in a world where assertive men are 'confident' and assertive women are 'bossy.' Maledoms fit into the status quo. Femdoms challenge it.

7.2.2.5 Clothes Make the Femdom

Men can be dominant in their tighty-whities. But a woman in colorful socks and comfy jeans can't be dominant. She needs a leather catsuit and high heel boots and a whip she wields better than Indiana Jones.

This is related to...

7.2.2.6 All Doms Have Dungeons

You aren't a good d-type if you don't have an entire basement (or at least a walk-in closet) full of bondage furniture, sadistic implements, etc,. Again, there's a reason why in BDSM romance, even more than mainstream romance, the maledom (it's almost always a maledom, see above) is usually rich. If they weren't rich they couldn't afford membership in that swanky, ultra-private BDSM club. And they would never have their huge collection of very expensive toys and tools.

Clothes and equipment don't make the d-type. And there is a huge tradition of do-it-yourself toys in kink communities. There are safety issues with some DIY (I've heard some nightmare stories about DIY fuck machines). But anyone who can make a bookshelf can make a spanking bench, belts work great for a spanking, and rope[20] and chains are available at any hardware store. Sure, the pretty leather cuffs are, well, *pretty*. But they aren't necessary, and lack of them doesn't make a dom any less domly.

7.2.2.7 I'm Sure I'm Forgetting Some

...but this covers the big ones. The ones you've probably heard or seen and may have internalized without noticing. Because fish don't notice the water. Hopefully, you'll be better able to recognize them—both in others and in yourself—going forward.

7.3 Recognizing Healthy and Unhealthy Power Exchange

It took a while, but by now you should know enough about kink that we're able to talk about healthy and unhealthy power exchange, and how you recognize them.

Hopefully, neither you nor anyone you know will ever end up in an unhealthy power exchange. But... it happens. It happens a lot. Sometimes because people don't know any better. Sometimes because people are abusers, users, and assholes.

So best to know what to look for.

Let's start with the big one—What does abuse look like in PE relationships?

7.3.1 Abuse in Power Exchange

As we covered back at the beginning, abuse is non-consensual control. Power exchange, as we know, involves consensual control. Sometimes, it can be hard to recognize the non-

---

20 If you buy rope that isn't intended for BDSM use, make sure you pick the right kind of fiber. And you'll need to look up how to care for it. Some types of rope at the hardware store aren't safe to use for bondage. Some others need to be treated before being safe.

consensual control of abuse in a power exchange dynamic.

We're going to take a look at some of the ways abuse can happen in power exchange and how to recognize it.

7.3.1.1 Kink-Based Abuse

Most abuse in the Scene follows the same patterns as vanilla abuse. There is one side of kinky abuse that vanilla folks won't have heard of: the abuser controlling the victim's kinks and kink expression.

Kink takes a lot of forms. It's common for folks who, on the surface, look compatible, actually not be compatible. For instance, a dominant and submissive may have different ideas about what dominance and submission look like.

In healthy kink, they either compromise or accept they are incompatible and look for other partners. But the kink-based abuser will try to force their partner into becoming what they want in a kinky partner. They may not abuse in the 'usual' manners. They may not cut their partner off from friends or family, may not try to control the finances so their partner can't escape, etc. (Though they will try to control their partner's access to the kink community!)

Because they aren't interested in that kind of control. They just want their partner to do kink right, damnit! (Or so they tell themselves.)

Which doesn't make it any less abusive. Or any less damaging.

And vanilla folk's view of kink (see: those myths we talked about) often means the victim actively hides everything from non-kinky friends and family. So other people aren't as likely to see the signs of abuse. Or be able to offer any useful help if they did.

7.3.1.2 50 Shades of Abuse

Seriously, this book is an amazing primer for what unsubtle abuse looks like in power exchange. I mean... there is nothing subtle about the abuse here. It's right there, from the stalking, to the ignoring her safeword, to the BS contract which he treats as a binding thing that she isn't allowed to break. (It wasn't and she was.)

But for the folks wise enough to avoid those books, let's take a more straightforward (and shorter!) look at obvious abuse in power exchange.

1. Ignoring safewords (this should go without saying. Ignoring

safewords is violating consent, we get this right?)

2. Breaking hard limits at all

3. Breaking soft limits when the person whose limit it is hasn't initiated/requested the activity

– this one may need some explanation because soft limits aren't a common concept in polyamory (IMO, it should be!) A soft limit is something that is an automatic 'no' about 99% of the time. BUT! you might like to try it, or you enjoy it when you are in the right mood, or you will do it once in a blue moon because your partner enjoys it. The default position on a soft limit is a 'no.' It only becomes a 'yes' if the person whose limit it is explicitly says 'let's do this.'

4. Badgering or harassing or guilting someone into changing their limits.

5. Trying to impose control outside of agreed-upon areas.

– saying yes to kissing doesn't mean you've said yes to sex. We all know this, right? Well, saying yes to a partner taking control of what you wear doesn't mean they get to control who your friends are.

6. Unilaterally initiating power exchange without the other person's agreement.

There's a pattern here, and it's a pretty clear one. Violating consent to make someone do something they haven't agreed to is abuse. (And in any case where violating consent isn't abuse—it's still violating consent and you shouldn't do it.)

Unfortunately, as obvious as these consent violations should be, a lot of people will excuse them when done by a d-type because 'it's D/s!' And when an s-type does it (Were you picturing the abuser as a d-type? Most people do. Go back and read over that list. There is nothing on it that is exclusive to d-types.) folks tend to miss it. Even in healthy power exchange s-types can look a stereotypical abuse victim—and nothing like the stereotype of an abuser.

7.3.1.3 Abusive S-types

I want to focus on abusive s-types for a minute, simply because so few people expect it. In the Scene, there are lots of warnings and talks and advice and etc about avoiding an abusive d-type. Crickets on avoiding abusive s-types.

I mentioned earlier that at one time I had started 'funishment' play with a sub when we hadn't discussed it beforehand. What happened that night was I told them to stay still while I fondled them. They couldn't hold perfectly still (duh!), and so I started talking about them being a 'bad' sub and needing to punish them. They put a stop to the scene. I did my best to give the aftercare they needed and reassure them that it was just play, I didn't think they were a bad sub, etc. All in all, it was your textbook 'oops, someone fucked up' scene that stops before it goes into harmful territory.

Well, that ended up being my introduction to abusive subs. See, I made a mistake, yeah. But they couldn't let the mistake go. By the end of that night, they had me in tears multiple times and begging them to please forgive me, give me another chance, etc. And it came up several more times over the next few weeks. They saw how I was beating myself up over that mistake and they used that against me.

With some exceptions, when an s-type is abusive it will be emotional and psychological abuse. Negging, gaslighting, etc.

Like all such abusers, they look for insecurities. If you are a new d-type and not yet confident in your dominance, you are their preferred target. But they will go after experienced and confident d-types as well. We all have insecurities that an abuser can latch onto and use to get into our heads and fuck us up.

A few things to watch for:

1. An s-type who tries to tell you how to be a d-type. This can be as blatant as 'if you were a real d-type you'd... (know how to do this, not make mistakes, wear a leather catsuit, etc, etc). But it can be subtle too.

2. An s-type who holds your mistakes over you and/or guilts you and makes you feel like a horrible person because of mistakes. (You are human. You will make mistakes, especially when you are new. A mistake doesn't make you a bad d-type, or a horrible person. A mistake doesn't mean you owe your s-type more than you would owe anyone else—that is, address and do what you can to correct the harm done and an effort to make sure it can't happen again, and an apology.)

3. An s-type who starts 'submitting' before you've agreed to power exchange and/or insists on submitting in areas you haven't agreed to take control in.

– Scarily, many people tell malesubs who want to introduce power exchange to stealth-submit. That is, start acting submissive to their significant other without talking about BDSM. Supposedly the SO will realize how wonderful it is to have the malesub doing everything they want and embrace their (usually her) inner dom. I could write a whole chapter on the problems with this scenario.[21]

1. S-Type Kink-Based Abuse

In my experience (which is another way of saying 'anecdotally') many abusive s-types whose abuse is kink-based would do better IDing as d-type bottoms. Basically, they want the scene to go the way they think it should go. But they want to be the one tied up and beaten and humiliated and so on and so forth.

They don't recognize that they want to control the scene, because they've bought the bottom=sub kool-aid. So they id as subs hoping to get their kink on and then try to force their d-type into doing scenes *their* way. They'd do a lot less harm if they admitted that they're dominant bottoms and went looking for service tops.

7.3.1.4 What to Look For

Recognizing abuse in PE can be harder than in non-PE relationships because most folks looking for abuse look for signs of *control*. That doesn't help much in power exchange relationships.

But there are still signs to look for, in your own relationship or others.'

Cutting off kink support

Abusers in kink relationships don't always try to cut their victims off from vanilla friends and family. Unless the victim is 'out' about being kinky, they have their own reasons to keep quiet about what goes on in the relationship.

But abusers will often cut a victim off from the kink community, refuse to let them read books about kink, and otherwise deny them a chance to learn more or connect with other kinky folks. They insist that you don't need to attend a munch/read a book/go on Fetlife/etc, they can teach you everything you need to know. This is an immediate red flag.

At best, they are one-twue-way assholes who don't want you to do kink differently than their twueism. At worst, they are abusers cutting you off from support and folks who might

---

21   There is a difference between a malesub in a vanilla a relationship *doing what his partner asks* and a malesub *tricking their partner into a dominant role*. If you do what your partner asks as an expression of your submissive nature that's fine, that's you being you. Doing what they ask as a way to sneak D/s into your relationship is *not* fine. That's being a manipulative and abusive asshole. Even more so when you start abdicating from decision making or refusing to give opinions in order to force them to 'take control.'

recognize the abuse.

Limit violations

You'd think this would be obvious, but too often an abuser can find ways to make a limit violation their victim's fault. There is no excuse for violating someone's kink limits. Anyone who makes excuses rather than apologizing and promising to not let it happen again/do their best to keep it from happening again is waving a red flag in your face. (Yes, accidents happen. If it is an accident, you should get an immediate apology and commitment ot make sure it doesn't happen again. If you don't, that's not abuse, but it is a major red flag.)

Refusing to renegotiate

Far too often 'you agreed to X' is held over your head as a tool of nonconsensual control. It doesn't matter what you agreed to, what you signed, how long the agreement has been in place. You can always say, 'Sorry, but I can't do that anymore. I'm calling 'Red' (or appropriate safeword) on your refusal to renegotiate. I'll see you again on the fourth of *Never*.'

Ignoring safewords

There is even less excuse for ignoring safewords than there is for violating limits. We can all get forgetful sometimes. And when you have multiple partners, keeping track of which limit goes with who can be overwhelming. (Which is why you should review your partners' limits from time to time to help you remember, yes?)

But there is no excuse for forgetting that *red means stop*. Or asparagus means stop. Or whatever safeword you are using. (Okay, if it's your first time using a new non-stoplight safeword, forgetting can happen. But red means stop? Come on.)

Using 'twueisms' to pressure you into changing

'A real dom would do...' 'If you aren't willing to push your limits you aren't a real sub.' 'How can you be a little if you won't wear a diaper?'

Especially if you have insecurities, abusers will leverage 'twueisms' to control you. Mostly, this type of control is kink-related. But it can be part of non-kink control as well. 'A good dom wouldn't let me drive, they'd take me where I need to go.' 'A well-behaved sub would quit their job and stay home to take care of me.'

Remember: YKINMK. And anyone who tries to force, shame, coerce, or badger you into doing kink (or anything else) in a way you don't like, is not a good person to be with.

7.4 Other Unhealthy Power Exchange

Someone made a comment on my blog once, equating my saying 'X isn't abusive' with 'any relationship that isn't abusive is healthy.'

And... no. Just... no.

Relationships can be unhealthy in lots of different ways. And most of them *aren't* abusive.

If you don't trust each other, that's unhealthy. (Especially in power exchange, for goodness' sake!)

If you don't talk to each other about problems and can't work together to solve them, that's unhealthy.

If *outside circumstances* make you feel trapped in this relationship, no matter how good to you your partner is, that's unhealthy.

We get this right? I've got a dead horse here and can move on? Good.

(I swear, I've had more dead horses in this book than in the last three put together. I'm not sure if I've changed that much, or if kink is just more prone to dead horses... But for all the weird shit I've seen in play parties and kink relationships, a horse head in the bed has never been one of them.)

7.4.1 Excessive Selfishness

A certain amount of selfishness is not only good, it is necessary. But even more so than most relationships, PE doesn't work if you aren't giving focus and attention to the other person. A vanilla monogamous couple can live parallel lives, only coming together to sleep and maybe for a few meals. It's not a relationship most people today would want, but it can be done without being unhealthy.

In power exchange that flat out won't work.

But even worse, some people try to make the power exchange all about them. A dom who only cares about their pleasure, and not about their sub. A little who only cares about getting taken care of and doesn't care about the needs or limits of their Adult. So on and so forth.

Power exchange is a commitment to, in different ways, take care of each other. Someone who is only in it for what they can get out of it makes it unhealthy real fast.

7.4.2 Can't Separate Reality from Fantasy

Unfortunately, some folks in kink think real relationships should look like fantasies—either their own, or books they've read. This overlaps heavily with twueism. A lot of these folks believe that (for instance) a twue d-type will always be in control, never need help and support, etc.

But it can take other forms as well. For instance, a person who thinks you can dive right into power exchange without negotiating or even getting to know each other. They will insist that an s-type begin deferring to them immediately. Or that a d-type should make them submit. Or begin 'submitting' without asking if the d-type wants their submission!

And, look, from a power exchange perspective, having someone who is exactly your type come up, grab your chin and say, 'You will call me 'Mistress.' ' or gracefully kneel before you and murmur, 'How may I serve you, Master?' is hot.

But it's a fantasy. That's not how relationships work.

(Okay, that can be how scenes at *some* play parties work, but only because the rules are laid out ahead of time. Everyone knows that any dom present can demand the service of any sub. Showing up is consenting to the rules of the game. But that's a scene at a party, not a relationship.)

It's easy enough to recognize this attitude when you first start talking with someone. But sometimes it can crop up unexpectedly mid-relationship.

7.5 So What Does Healthy Power Exchange Look Like?

Healthy power exchange is fulfilling and satisfying for all parties. That's not to say folks in healthy power exchange are always happy and giddy or whatever. Life happens, even to people in perfect relationships. But the stuff upsetting folks in healthy power exchange will be financial problems, or medical shit, or the kid not doing well in school. If you've been together long enough to be past NRE and still usually smile when talking about your partner(s), anticipate the next scene you do together, etc., you are okay.

Another thing to look for is communication. Specifically communication about problems. Is everyone comfortable saying 'hey, we need to talk about this?' For folks who can't be that direct (for whatever reason), are there means in place (a journal, a note box, etc) that they can use? Are everyone's concerns respected and listened to?

8 Kink and Polyamory – When You Want to Explore Kink

We've talked about kink, and what you can expect when other folks in your polycule are doing kinky stuff. If you're interested in kinky stuff yourself, this chapter is for you.

8.1 Is This Your Idea or Someone Else's?

In the big picture it doesn't matter if trying kink if your idea or someone else's. However, it can make some difference, especially in the beginning.

If it's your idea, then you probably have an idea of what roles and scenes you might like to try. You're going in seeking stuff for you that you know you are into. If someone else suggested kink, then they likely have things that they would like you to do, and you may have no idea what you would be into.

You need to have room to explore. Your partner may be looking for a dom, but that doesn't mean *you* fit that role. And if you don't fit that role, it doesn't mean you aren't kinky. Don't be afraid to try other roles, other places you can fit.

Also—remember that abusers will use introducing kink as a means of control. Your partner needs to be supporting your kinky exploration. They especially should be introducing you to other people/resources you can learn from. Not forcing you into their idea of what kink, and your role in kink, should look like.

8.2 Finding Your Roles and Kinks

We covered the main 'roles' in kink earlier, but let's take another look now to make sure they are fresh in your mind:

Top: is the active participant in a kink scene

Verse: someone who tops and bottoms

Bottom: is the passive or receptive participant in a kink scene

Dom: takes control of the sub in a power exchange

Switch: someone who can dom or sub

Sub: gives control to the dom during a power exchange

Most other kink roles are sub-headings of these six. A rigger is a rope top. A rope slut or rope bunny is a rope bottom. A sadist is a pain play top, a masochist is a pain play bottom.

You get the idea.

The best way to know for sure that a role suits you is to try it. But, honestly, start with your imagination.[22]

Read a description of a kink scene. (You can find thousands on Literotica or Fetlife, never mind all the personal kink blogs scattered around the internet). Can you picture yourself in that scene? Do you imagine yourself as the top or bottom, dom or sub?

Once you've read or watched a good range of scenes, try imagining your ideal scene. Does it involve rope? Pain? Blindfolds? Just bodies and obedience?

Those endless BDSM checklists come in handy here. What makes you lick your lips and start fantasizing? What squicks you? What sounds like it might be interesting but you aren't sure?

When you get a chance, try some of it. Some folks start out trying a few things and exploring those few things fully before trying something else on their list.

Others try a bit of this today and a bit of that tomorrow. Once they've tried everything they can right now, they decide what (if anything) they want to focus on for the time being.

Early on, lack of equipment will be a major restriction. You can't use leather cuffs that you don't have, never mind big things like spanking benches or fuck machines.

Actually, lack of equipment will likely be an issue throughout your entire kinky experience. As mentioned earlier, most folks can't afford the kinky supply room/dungeon seen in BDSM

---

22 Meg-John Barker and Justin Hancock's Understanding Ourselves Through Erotic Fantasies Zine might be helpful if you can get a copy.

romance novels.

But pervertables[23][24] are a thing, as is DIY kinky crafting. There is a large DIY and pervertable community within the Scene, and lots of folks willing to help you learn what's what.

Still, some things—including pervertables and DIY stuff—is best to wait on until you can learn a bit. Using the wrong thing as a pervertable can be an invitation for an infection or hospital visit.

8.3 Connecting with Community

For several reasons—we've covered most of them already— connecting with other kinky folks is very important.

The two main practical reasons are:

1. Learning how to do kink safely

2. Having folks you can talk about kink with who can warn you if they see a red flag on the kink side of your relationship

That said, for most of us the real main reason is it's fun talk kink with other kinky folks.

But how do you connect with other kinky folks?

8.3.1 Where to Find Kinksters

Of course, it helps to know where to look for kinksters. Here are a few suggestions to get you started.

8.3.1.1 Fetlife

Fetlife is the kink community clearinghouse these days. There are a lot of legit criticisms of the site, but it really has become the Facebook of kink. (With fewer privacy issues.) Cutting yourself off from Fet is cutting yourself off from a lot of the Scene.

Fet has groups for every type of kink you can imagine, and many you probably can't.

Whatever the site's other flaws, Baku has done a very good job of keeping Fet from turning into another dating site. That

---

23 Normal household items used in a 'perverted' way. Cucumbers are a classic example of a pervertable.

24 Yes, I said 'improvising sex toys bad' in Safer Sex. The kink community has decades of experience in *safely* improvising. Tap that expertise before doing turning random household item *a* into a pervertable. You don't want to find out the hard way that shampoo makes very bad lube.

doesn't mean folks won't solicit or send dick pics or whatever. Humans on the internet are, well, humans on the internet. For good or ill. But you can always set your location to Antarctica. I swear in the world according to Fetlife, Antarctica has a bigger population than NYC.

The 'Ask a ______' groups are great places to go to, well, ask stuff. Go to Ask a Submissive if you have questions about being a new submissive, what submissives are looking for, etc.

Fetlife is also a good place to look for local groups.

8.3.1.2 Local Sex Shop

Some local sex shops will hold workshops and classes by kink experts. They usually know where the local munch is and who to get in touch with to get an invite. And if there is a club or dungeon in the area, they'll probably know about it.

Buyer beware, not everyone talking kink at a sex shop knows what they are talking about. And that can include the folks giving workshops. If a workshop is being offered, it can be a good idea to google the presenter and check their experience and reputation.

8.3.1.3 Social Media

There are active BDSM communities on Twitter, Facebook, and Reddit. The community on Tumblr got hit hard by the Pornocalypse when Verizon bought Yahoo. But the part of the kink community there is still holding on. Fediverse has some kink-dedicated instances and a lot of kink-friendly instances. Instagram has a very active rope scene and many sex workers, sexy/kinky events, and venues with accounts.

Hashtags: #kink #BDSM #bondage and many others.

8.3.1.4 Your Local Polyam Meetup or Favorite Polyam Forum

As mentioned elsewhere, the Venn diagram of polyam folks and kinky folks has a pretty big overlap. In some places, you can ask your local polyam meetup who's into kink and get responses from over half the group.

8.3.2 When You Can't People

Lots of folks can't people well. That is, can't handle interacting with other people or interact in a way that isn't accepted for reasons beyond our control. Often because of anxiety, autism, lack of accessibility, or other issues.

For folks who can't people, online interaction may be easier than in person, so check out the online options if you can. But if online doesn't work, you can still learn about kink. There are lots of books, blogs, and videos to help.

Or, hell, nothing stopping you from joining Fetlife and being a lurker.

A few suggestions to get you started:

Conquer Me by Kacie Cunningham

Sharyn Ferns' books and blog (https://www.domme-chronicles.com/)

Stabbity's Blog Not Just Bitchy (http://notjustbitchy.com/ no longer updated, but awesome stuff in the archives)

Sugarbutch Chronicles by Sinclair Sexsmith (http://www.sugarbutch.net/)

The Duchy (https://www.theduchy.com/)

BDSMCafe.com (https://bdsmcafe.com/)

Kink Academy (https://www.kinkacademy.com/)

Life, Leather and the Pursuit of Happiness by Steve Lenius

8.4 Your First Scene

If possible, plan your first scene with an experienced kinkster who you know and trust. It's generally a good idea to keep the first scene short—around 15 minutes is good. Have a clear idea of what to expect. What activities are on the table? What are you supposed to do during the scene?

Oh, I don't mean there can't be spontaneity. Of course, if you are subbing then you aren't going to know ahead of time everything the dom will do or order. But what ever role your taking, you should know the basics. For instance, this is going to be a rope-and-flogging scene where you will be the bottom and exploring bondage and pain play.

Or this will be a fully clothed service scene where you will be the dom and ordering the sub to do basic care tasks for you (make tea, foot massage, etc).

For after the scene, make sure you have some basic care supplies on hand. A warm blanket, water, Gatorade, or your 'I need a pick-me-up' drink of choice, a high energy snack, your favorite book, etc.

You aren't likely to need much aftercare doing a short intro scene, but sometimes the first time hits people hard. So be prepared.

If you are playing at an event, don't be afraid to let the dungeon monitors know that you are new and might need some help. That's what they are there for, and there is nothing to be ashamed of.

Finally (and most importantly), your first kink scene can be much like the first sexual experience. There will likely be awkwardness. And fumbling. And moments where you feel absolutely ridiculous. And that is all okay. Be prepared to feel silly calling your top 'sir.' To worry like you look ridiculous wielding a flogger while wearing clogs. To flub something up so you end up sprawled on the floor and wondering how you got there.

If you can laugh about it, all the better. We've all been there. New things are new.

8.5 Kink Is for Everyone—But Some of Us Have Extra Needs

I've tried to be inclusive throughout this book. Hopefully, I don't need to say 'yes, people with disabilities, chronic illnesses, or recovering from trauma can be kinky.' (But, just in case, there it is.)

And (duh) having kids doesn't stop you from being kinky. Nor does being a teenager or an elder. But being one or more of those can create some extra requirements. So we're going to spend a few minutes talking about those.

8.5.1 Kink and Disability/Chronic Illness

Yes, you absolutely can be a dom in a wheelchair. Or a sub.

And depression doesn't mean you can't love rope or chains. Fibro means you need to be careful how you kink, not that you can't kink.

Disability and chronic illnesses vary too widely for me to say anything that would be universally applicable here. But don't be afraid to be creative. If you can't fit in the popular idea and expectation of a given kink role, you can still do it. You just need to think outside the box.

It will likely take some time to figure out how best to adapt your kink to your needs. It's okay to lean heavily on the community here. Folks have been doing kink with disability and chronic illness for decades. No need to reinvent the wheel, learn from those of us who've been there.

One very important thing—if your stuff has an impact on your ability to communicate with others, whether you are Deaf, autistic, prone to panic attacks, whatever, make doubly sure your kink partners know that. Have a plan in place for if you need to tell them something beyond what the current scene allows for. This can be relying on safewords, setting up a signal set, or even your partner learning your language and/or body language. (Hey, a speaking partner of a deaf person can learn sign language, right? If not fully fluent than at least basic pidgin.) Whatever your situation or needs, keeping communication going is very important to safety and meeting everyone's needs.

8.5.2 Kink and Trauma

We've established that people aren't kinky because of abuse. But trauma, both from abuse and from other stuff, can have pretty far-reaching and (sometimes) weird interactions with kink.

For a personal example—there's a reason I don't submit. On my own, without the impact of my trauma, I'd probably be a vers switch instead of a vers dom. In fact, I used to submit all the time.

Eventually, though, I realized that when I submit I fall into a very unhealthy headspace. Even for a short scene, I fall into a Stolkholm-syndrome-like headspace where I lose track of my safety, limits, and needs. Everything becomes about pleasing my dom so they don't hurt me. Even to the point of self-harm. Even if the dom is someone who has my complete trust.

Yeah, I don't do that anymore. My trauma put some deep scars in my psyche that make submitting flat out unsafe.

On the other hand, (I don't know how much this relates to my trauma, but I have some guesses) rope is absolutely my safe space. Nothing feels better on a stressed-out day than wrapping myself in a big rope and letting it hold me safe. If I have a partner doing fun stuff to me at the same time, so much the better.

Some folks who have been through trauma have found pain-play to be helpful. The pain takes them to a headspace where they can release the built-up tension and mental toxins that they haven't yet learned to release in daily life.

I've known folks who used rape play as a way to process and heal from actual rape they've lived through.

On the other hand, sometimes a kink scene can hit triggers and re-traumatize someone because of its similarity to old trauma.

One of these days someone needs to write an entire book on kink and trauma. Preferably a kinky someone with a psych degree who has lived through trauma themselves.

The point here is that if you have lived through trauma, it may interact with kink in weird ways that would never have guessed or expected. Make sure your partners know any potential triggers, know (and use!) your safeword. And when trying something new, keep the aftercare kit handy and your support network on speed dial.

8.5.3 Parenting and Kink

Someone compiled list of ridiculous 'slave rules' recently. One rule was that said slaves should always go naked. Apparently, the rule writer thought that BDSM slaves can't be parents. Or hold jobs, for that matter.

You'll see this thinking a lot, unfortunately. Folks talk about kink, and power exchange especially, as if all kinksters exist in a world where there are only adults. No infants requiring care or kids popping out of bed in the middle of the night because they had a nightmare.

Partly this is concern that talking about parenting while kinky will lead to assumptions and accusations. People claiming you are exposing kids to sex stuff or are a child abuser. Part of it is enjoying the fantasy of kink without real-life restrictions and forgetting the difference between fantasy and reality.

Bedroom-only kink when you are a parent is no different than having vanilla sex when you are a parent. You do your thing behind closed doors. You keep the lube/condoms/sex toys/rope tucked away somewhere the kids aren't likely to find it. You try to have your fun when the kids are asleep or other times when they aren't likely to interrupt.

If they see something, you deal with it as best you can, like any other sex stuff. Kid walked in on me one time doing some self-breast-bondage. He asked what I was doing. I said it was sex stuff, and therefore none of his business. He was supposed to be in bed. He asked how it was sex stuff; I said, we'll discuss that when you are older, now back to bed.

End of discussion, end of the issue.

In hindsight, I should also have reminded him to knock before opening doors.

Probably best to save the scenes with loud stuff (assuming

you kink that way) for when the kids aren't around.

For power exchange outside the bedroom, well, most of that isn't sex. There's no inherent reason you can't do it around the kids. Most PE parents develop approaches that look vanilla. After all, there's nothing noticeably kinky about saying 'Yes dear' when your spouse or significant other asks you to do something.

Some folks choose to be open about their power exchange with their kids. This can be very straightforward 'we've agreed that [parent] is in charge because that works for us. Some families have one parent in charge because that works for those parents. In other families, no one person is in charge and the parents make decisions together. Other families have other ways of doing things.'

'Nuff said.

8.5.3.1 Parents Looking for Kinky Partners

Unfortunately, some folks aren't willing to accept that your kids come first. It happens in polyamory and vanilla dating and it can definitely happen in kink. So if you are looking for out of the bedroom power exchange and are a parent, you may run into some twuist assholes. Folks who act like your being a parent means you can't be a real d-type or s-type.

Don't be afraid to make your kids and their needs part of your limits and boundaries. Whether it's 'no kink around the kids' or 'I have to be home every night to cook dinner,' your need to be a good parent is always valid. Anyone who doesn't respect that is someone you don't need in your life.

8.5.4 Teens and Kink

It isn't uncommon for folks to realize they are kinky while they are still in teenagers. If you are a teen kinkster, you will have a lot of trouble finding places where you can learn and explore. Sex stuff is intertwined with kink, and no one wants to risk being accused of grooming you for rape or assault or whatever else.

That doesn't mean you can't start learning. Some places with a large kink population will have teen munches. The Scarleteen website has some info on kink, including kink with disability. (http://scarleteen.com/)

If you want to explore kink with other teens, have fun (safely). I highly recommend you avoid kinky relationships with legal adults, especially folks much older than you. First, because there are predators who will take advantage of your interest in kink. Second, because your parents/teachers/etc are way more likely to go after a *kinky* adult partner than a vanilla adult partner. So you can be putting them at risk as well as yourself.

Blindfolds, bedroom-only PE, light bondage, pet play without gear, openhanded spankings, and non-pain sensation play are all things you can explore with little risk. And without doing any sex stuff unless you want to.

8.5.5 Elders and Kink

If you are an elder, you know better than I do that getting old often means acquiring health problems and frailties that aren't health problems yet. Your skin likely gets damaged easily. You'll bruise more than when you were younger. So extra care with bondage and impact play is important.

But that doesn't mean you can't kink. Just like folks with disabilities and chronic illnesses, know your limits and communicate them to anyone you play with.

If you are showing any signs of dementia, talk with someone in your family, polycule, or care team you trust about your interest in kink. They can help you explore safely and ensure you are making good decisions for you and your partners.

8.6 Talking with Your Partners

It's a personal call whether you tell the folks in your polycule that you are exploring kink or not. If there is a specific partner you want to explore kink with, of course, you need to talk with them. And it's helpful if your other partners are likely to notice changes in your interactions with your kinky partner (for instance, if you are doing 24/7 power exchange). You should probably say something if it will impact your interactions with the rest of the polycule.

But... it isn't necessary even then. You don't necessarily owe anyone an explanation as long as you are keeping your commitments and respecting limits and boundaries.

If you want to tell your polycule, how you do it is again, personal, but the culture of your polycule is definitely a factor. For instance, if your polycule tends to have a big sit down discussion from time to time, that's a good time to bring it up. If you don't have a custom of that kind of round table, then talking with people one-on-one might work better.

If the rest of the polycule is also new to kink, you may need to explain. Or, you know, get them a copy of this book.

8.7 Adding 24/7 Power Exchange to Your Polycule

How adding power exchange to your polycule will impact things varies. Largely, it depends on how entwined you and your power exchange partner(s) are with the rest of the polycule. It also depends on how intense a power exchange you are doing. For instance, in parallel polyamory, starting a bedroom-only power exchange won't affect anyone else in the polycule. At least, not any more than getting a new job or a new partner. Schedules might shift, you might need to set some new limits with your other partners. But no big.

On the other hand, if you do tight kitchen table polyamory or (even more so) have a group living situation, adding power exchange can have a large impact. Especially 24/7 power exchange. Your other partners will likely see the change in how you and your power exchange partner(s) interact. More, that change will likely impact the dynamic of the group as a whole. The more intense the power exchange, the more impact it will have.

8.7.1 Making Adjustments

You and your partner(s) who are starting power exchange will likely have new boundaries based on the power exchange. The s-type(s) new boundaries will be based on the orders given by the d-type(s). However many folks don't realize that the d-type(s) will have new boundaries as well—boundaries based on their responsibilities to the s-type(s).

If those new boundaries can impact other folks in the polycule, you should probably be communicating them to everyone else, yes? Examples might be 'I will be in bed by 10pm each night' or 'I need to have time Sunday to pick out s-type's clothes for the week.'

And don't forget:

When the d-type is setting rules (and taking on responsibilities) they/you need to remember everyone else's boundaries. You might want to explore chastity and orgasm control. Good for you. But doing so might mean the other folks in the polycule will need the d-type's okay for certain sex stuff with the s-type.[25] That would violate a lot of polyam folk's boundaries.

---

25 Might. Depends on how you do it. If Erin is locked in a chastity device all week and Lorrin has the key, that has a clear impact on what other people can do with Erin.

Of course, you can violate boundaries if you want. That's also a reality of boundaries. But even if you are okay being shitty to your partners, you'll still need to deal with the consequences. And, you know, try *talking* with your partners and metamours? Maybe they'd be okay with skipping sex for a week so you can explore chastity, as long as they get the respect of being asked first.

8.7.2 Mixing Egalitarian Polyamory and Power Exchange

Egalitarian polyamory and power exchange can work very well together. The key is that egalitarian polyamory is about all *relationships* being equal. In egalitarian polyamory, no relationship has power over other relationships. Power exchange is between individuals, not relationships.

Here's an easy way to make it work:

Your power exchange can have a clear limit—the d-type can make no rules that will impact people outside the power exchange without their consent.

For instance, the chastity example earlier would not be allowed.

However, it could be argued the other way. If Danny and Ayda want chastity in their power exchange, then why should Idris get to veto that? If Danny decided on his own that he wanted to wear a chastity device, would Idris get a say? Nope. So why do they get a say here?

I would argue that both views are valid. I tend to come down more on one side myself, and that's come out in this book. But if you come down on the other side that's okay. What's important is that your polycule agrees on which view y'all will be working from.

Having said that, I'm going to expand on that second view a bit. It's another one of those areas that folks might need to lean in on.

Doing something that impacts another relationship isn't the same as having power over another relationship. If my nesting partner gets a new job, that's going to impact the rest of my relationships because it will change my availability. Both my schedule and my available spoons will change. That doesn't

Me, I'd skip the chastity and just tell pet that she wasn't allowed to orgasm without permission. Then pet can continue as-usual with her other partners, and if she can't keep from orgasming… then I get *my* fun.

mean other people have a say over my nesting partner's job, right?

But stuff like jobs, medical shit, everyone (who has a realistic view of relationships) knows that stuff can change. And knows that jobs, medical shit, etc, can impact other relationships. Being in a relationship with someone nonmonogamous is consenting to some of those impacts. But consent requires *knowledge*. With kink, and especially power exchange, many folks don't know what the possible impacts are. They can't consent to them as part of the relationship.

Which brings us back to what?

Communication.

Make sure your non-PE partners know about the possible impacts power exchange can have. Give them a chance to give *informed* consent and set boundaries based on knowledge.

8.7.2.1 Group Decision Making

This one is for out-of-the-bedroom PE.

If your polycule does any level of group decision making, it's important to think about how your PE will impact that. For a simple example—many power exchange relationships include food controls. Sometimes for the fun of it, sometimes as part of the d-type helping the s-type meet certain health goals. How will other folks feel if the s-type doesn't 'get' a vote on where to go for dinner? Or the d-type effectively gets two votes—the s-types and their own?

Of course, power exchange can also impact much more weighty decisions, like living arrangements, which other partners might be more concerned about.

Again, you can keep the power exchange from impacting these decisions. Either by not giving the d-type power over areas that your polycule decides as a group, or by suspending the power exchange during group decisions.

Some folks want that level of power exchange. And you can have it. But make sure you talk with your other partners and let them know that this is how you and your PE partners will be doing things. Don't be afraid to remind then choice involves being able to *not* choose. If someone not in a power exchange said 'whatever X person wants,' would they say 'you can't do that, you have to choose!' I'm guessing not.

But not everyone will be comfortable with it. So again, let everyone else know the deal so they can be prepared and can set any boundaries they feel they need to.

8.7.3 Sometimes a Polycule Becomes a Household or Staircase

No one in my polycule set out to build a Household or Staircase (currently staircase, but probably going to end up with a full household set up). We fell into it because, it turns out, most of us are kinky. Michael, Michon and I started (separately) in vanilla relationships, talked about our kinks, started with bedroom stuff, and ended up in 24/7 PE. Everyone Michael and I have gotten involved with since we got together has known we were kinky. And that we were open to power exchange. At this point, I only know of one person in the entire network who isn't kinky and involved in PE (some folks are bedroom only) and he's said he might want to explore it. So... yeah. It's a thing.

LGBT folks and geeks and metalheads seem to end up finding each other and forming a social group whether they intend to or not. Well, it happens with kinky folks too. And when your whole polycule is kinky and into PE, you can end up with your entire polycule being part of a power exchange network as well.

If it happens and everyone's happy with it, great!

If it doesn't happen or you don't want it to happen, that's okay. You do what's right for you. In kink *and* polyamory.

If it's a goal for you, we're back to: communicate, damnit! (And you maybe making some hard decisions.)

8.8 Wrapping Up

That covers all the basics. Obviously, the devil is in the details and you'll do a lot of work sorting out those details.

I'm not getting into how to find a kinky partner or what to do in your kink relationships. There's tons of kink-specific resources, most of which will work fine for polyam folks. I'm gonna wrap up with some general info that might be useful— common terms we didn't cover in the book and that kind of thing. But before we do that, I want to touch on...

9 Edge cases

I originally had these in the section on healthy and unhealthy power exchange. But the thing is, they don't always involve power exchange. And really, they are things everyone dealing with kink should be aware of. These are the edge cases...

Edge cases is my term for some things that I, for one, can't say if they are healthy are not. These edge cases are hotly debated in the Scene. You'll need to make your own judgments. But I suggest not getting involved in any of these without a lot of thought and discussion with people you trust.

9.1 Kink in Public

For the most part, we've been looking at what is healthy for the people in the relationship. But relationships affect people around them too.

So what about taking your kink in public?

9.1.1 Being Yourself

Some kinks can be in public without being noticed. Many power exchange folks have found ways to be subtle. For instance, the s-type saying 'yes love' instead of 'yes mistress.' Or wearing necklace-collars.

But some folks choose to be openly kinky. For instance, including humiliation play in their evening at a restaurant. Or an s-type kneeling next to their d-type while waiting at the bus stop.

Is this okay? What impact does it have on people around you? Do you care?

Most kinky folks agree that somethings are okay—saying 'yes

master' outs yourself but doesn't harm or inconvenience anyone else. Grabbing your partner and slamming them into the wall may be a fun kink at home. In public, folks watching will think it's assault. Some might try to intervene and it might be a trigger for abuse survivors who see you. Less of an issue but still out there is 'benign' obvious stuff. Doing humiliation play like having a bottom wear a pig snout and eat with their mouth while oinking can be rather freaky for the vanilla folks around you.

Everyone will have their own idea of what is okay in public and what should be kept in private. But being obvious about your kink is definitely an edge thing.

9.1.2 Exhibitionism

It's a whole 'nother thing when you aren't just being yourself in public but *getting off on* folks seeing your kink. Most kinky folks think exhibitionist kink or sex in public is a consent issue. It's also illegal in many places. Keep it to play parties and such where folks have consented to your getting off on them watching.

But it can be argued the other way—you aren't involving other folks, interacting with them or expecting them to do anything. As long as you are within the limits of the law (and/or custom) why would you need their consent to something you and your partner are doing?

You'll need to decide for yourself how you feel. But at the very least don't be an exhibitionist in public spaces without being sure it's something you are okay with—including the possible consequences.

9.2 Consensual Nonconsent

Consensual nonconsent, or con noncon, is when you agree that after a given point, the s-type or bottom cannot withdraw consent. Folks doing con noncon may have a safeword, but it doesn't stop the scene. It is for the s-type or bottom to signal that they need to say something that may change the d-type's mind about what they are doing. The d-type is not required or expected to end the scene.

Consensual nonconsent is something of a fraught topic in the Scene. Many people feel that you can't consent to a situation where your consent will be ignored or denied. Some folks feel it might be okay for a single scene. In a con noncon scene, folks negotiate everything beforehand, but during the scene itself the s-type or bottom doesn't get to safeword or 'tap out.' A few folks have embraced con noncon *relationships*. In noncon relationships, the s-type agrees to a life-long PE total-power exchange relationship with no renegotiation or limits. In this case, the s-type is almost always someone who identifies as a slave.

Honestly, con noncon is more talked about than done, but some folks do it. I had a chance once to talk with a self-identified slave in a con noncon relationship. She said that if she ever 'lost her mind' and wanted out of the relationship, her Master would chain her in the basement until she came to her senses. And her husband would help him.

Yeah, I... honestly, I'm fucking uncomfortable with that. And I expect most folks reading this are as well. But do I have the right to tell *her* that she shouldn't be in this relationship that makes her happy? Nonconsensual paternalism isn't a good look on anyone...

Anecdotally, fantasies of both con noncon and noncon are common, among kinky folks and the general population. So don't assume that someone who shares a noncon fantasy is into con noncon for real.

Similarly, rape play in the Scene is almost always role play with safewords and limits and everything. I've heard of plenty of people doing rape play. Only heard of one person who did it a con noncon way.

Short version: con noncon is a thing. Unless you get active in the Scene and various kink communities, you are unlikely to run into it. If you run into stuff that looks like noncon or con noncon, check in with people who are familiar with the situation first.

10 General Info that Might Be Useful

10.1 The Scene

Th e Scene (note the capital) is a term for kinky culture and society. Not all kinky folks consider ourselves part of the Scene. Many folks keep their kink as a personal preference. They don't go to play parties, join BDSM forums, etc. The kinkier you are, the more likely you are to be drawn into the Scene, however. In one way or another, the Scene is the only place to really learn about kink. That includes everything from safety practices to where to find a good leather collar.

10.1.1 Subspace/Domspace

It's pretty common in kink scenes for people to enter altered mental states. A lot of what I'm going to share in this section is speculative because as far as I know there hasn't been much science done on this.

It's generally agreed that chemicals play a large part in these altered mental states. Particularly: endorphins and adrenaline.[26]

Less talked about is how some kinks can have a meditative function. Complex rope work, in particular, is known to have a meditative effect. (For both sides of the rope.) Wielding the whip in a long flogging scene can be similarly meditative.

26 More information for those interested: *Between Pleasure and Pain: A Pilot Study on the Biological Mechanisms Associated With BDSM Interactions in Dominants and Submissives*, January 2020, Journal of Sexual Medicine, DOI: 10.1016/j.jsxm.2020.01.001

Finally, some level of sensory deprivation is common in kink play. This can range from mild (blindfold) to intense (full hood, vacuum beds).

In general discussion, folks don't attempt to differentiate the different types of altered mental states. It's all grouped together under 'subspace.' Occasionally someone will bring up 'domspace,' a reminder that it's not just subs that hit altered mental states. (Though pain play bottoms hit them more often than most. See: Endorphins and adrenaline.)

Healthy kink requires awareness and knowledge of your and your partners' mental state. Most of us enjoy going into our spaces, but altered mental states, even completely natural altered mental states, affect our judgment.

Many s-types and bottoms in subspace will lose some or all of their ability to communicate coherently. In deep, subspace someone may not be able to say a safeword–or remember one!

A d-type or top in domspace can lose track of how much they have done, leading to injury. Theirs or their partners. Sometimes both.

That's not to say that spaces should be avoided. But they are one reason a good top checks in throughout the scene. That's both self-checks and verbal checks on their bottom(s). It makes sure no one has gone so deep they lose track of safety.

Finally, getting into subspace or domspace often means that when you come out of it you are going to drop.

10.1.2 Edgeplay

Edgeplay refers particularly risky kinks. A few folks who've been around since the 80s have said that edgeplay used to only refer to the handful of kinks. Things that had a real risk of killing someone—like asphyxiation play. I don't remember the full list— it was four or five things really risky things. These days edgeplay has a more flexible usage. But it still means things that most kinksters (or at least, the speaker) won't try because of safety concerns.

Note: Stuff that isn't considered edgeplay can still be dangerous if done wrong.

Note two: *Edging* is unrelated to edgeplay and is usually part of orgasm denial. A generally safe, if incredibly frustrating, sexual kink.

10.1.3 Dungeons

A dungeon is any space dedicated to kinky activities. Some folks have a dungeon in their home, but most of us can't afford to set aside an entire room for kink. Kink clubs, public and private, may refer to their playroom as a dungeon.

10.1.4 Play Parties

A play party is an event where folks are meant to do kinky stuff. If there is one available, play parties will take place in a dungeon. But often it's 'just' a rented room at a local sex club/adult store for public play parties or someone's living room for private play parties.

10.1.5 Private Clubs

Most kinky clubs are members only. This is partly for safety and partly for privacy.

Having said this, while the kind of kink clubs you find in BDSM romance books may exist, I've never heard of one. Most kinksters can't afford to pay hundreds or thousands of dollars membership fees for a club. Which is what those extensive background checks, high tech security, full-time dungeon monitors, so on and so forth would cost. Never mind leather chairs, fancy carpeting, a raised stage for shows, etc, etc.

Much more common is a club that has a basic entrance interview, a couple of volunteers acting as dungeon monitors, a handful of pieces of homemade dungeon furniture, and a 'snack bar.' Said snack bar likely consists of bottled water, some fresh fruit, and a handful of chocolate bars for aftercare.

10.1.6 Munches

You may be familiar with munches from polyamory groups. Same basic deal. Kinky folks get together for a social event where folks (usually) keep their clothes on. It's a chance to hang out, meet other locals and talk kinky stuff with folks who understand. Where possible, groups will arrange a munch in a private location.

One munch I went to rented a room at the local VFW. (If you are unfamiliar, the VFW is a US veterans' organization. I admit I've often wondered if they knew exactly *who* they were renting too.) Because it was a private room in a private building, they were able to do presentations and educational workshops on different types of kinky play. They even brought in vendors with rope or toys a few times.

But it's more common for munches to meet at local

restaurants where that kind of thing wasn't possible.

10.1.7 DM

A DM or dungeon monitor is in charge of safety in a dungeon or play party. They keep an ear out for safewords, intervene in a scene that is becoming unsafe, make sure everyone is using equipment correctly, and generally keep everything in the playroom as safe as possible.

(Yes, if you are in a bunch of kinky D&D players this can get confusing.)

10.1.8 Fetlife

For better or worse (I have my own opinion), Fetlife has become the center of the kink community online. It's a social media/forum site for fetishists and kinky folks to connect, talk about kink, etc.

Unfortunately, the kink community is something of a victim of Fetlife's success. Fet is in many ways the Facebook of kink. It dominates the Scene—if you don't participate in Fet you are cut off from a lot of the Scene, offline as well as on. For instance, several times I needed to join a Fetlife group in order to join a local kink group. Doing it that way helps with privacy, but excludes folks who aren't on Fet.

Fetlife itself is a decent website, a bit too dominated by normative expectations. 90% of Kinky and Popular (the most popular posts on the site) are pictures of conventionally pretty white women. Usually in a submissive pose or tied up, but sometimes with nothing kinky in the pic.

That said, individual groups on Fet tend to have their own culture. I learned a lot on Fet and met a lot of great folks. Every couple of years I get tempted into reactivating my old account, maybe one of these days I'll stick around for a while.

10.1.9 CollarSpace

CollarSpace, formerly CollarMe, is/was the OKC of the kink world. It was also, at one time, a viable competitor with Fetlife as it had Forums and Chatrooms for members. Unfortunately, it's likely on its last legs. Not only has it closed down a lot of features, it's also redirecting people to sign up with Alt.com. I can't figure out how to make a new CollarSpace account anymore. A lot of kinky folks are used to giving out our CollarSpace info for other kinky folks to contact us... Sadly, it seems that won't be the way of the future.

10.1.10 Alt.com

I don't know much about this site. I've avoided it as one more annoying dating site that promises 'thousands of hot women in your area!' I'm including it here because CS is redirecting new folks to Alt. I expect this will be the new main home for kinky dating online.

I hope they add forums and chat rooms. I miss CS chat rooms.

10.1.11 Missing Stair Theory

Missing Stair Theory was first proposed by Cliff Pervocracy (who is absolutely worth reading if you can). You can find the original essay here: http://pervocracy.blogspot.com/2012/06/missing-stair.html.

"Have you ever been in a house that had something just egregiously wrong with it? Something massively unsafe and uncomfortable and against code, but everyone in the house had been there a long time and was used to it? 'Oh yeah, I almost forgot to tell you, there's a missing step on the unlit staircase with no railings. But it's okay because we all just remember to jump over it.'

"Some people are like that missing stair."

Cliff proposed Missing Stair Theory after learning about a known rapist in his community. Rather than confronting the rapist, everyone was trying to warn newcomers or babysit the rapist at play parties. Generally, they worked around the rapist rather than *fixing the problem*.

The term 'Missing Stair' has spread a fair bit in kink circles. Some polyamorous folks have started using it too.

10.1.12 Auctions

Sub/slave auctions do happen in the Scene, but again very little like what you'd read about in erotica. They're more like the Bachelor/Bachelorette auctions some places do for fundraisers. The winning d-type gets to play with the auctioned s-type for the evening, all the s-type's usual limits applying.

Local kink communities use auctions to fun and raise money. The money might go to support the local club/munch group/etc or for a charity.

The main difference between a kink auction and a Bachelor/Bachelorette auction is that Bachelor/Bachelorette auctions generally assume the winners and ah... prizes will go on a date somewhere else and somewhen else. Not the evening of the auction.

Most kink auctions take place at the local dungeon/kink club so the 'dates' can take place immediately. And observing the resulting public scenes (if any) can be part of the fun for the folks who don't take part in the auction or don't win their bids.

10.1.13 Contracts

Some polyam folks like to write up relationship agreements. Similarly, some kinky folks like to put their power exchange agreements on paper in a 'contract.'

To be clear—I don't know a single jurisdiction where a power exchange contract is legally enforceable. If you *want* a legally enforceable contract, talk with a lawyer and be prepared to be disappointed.

Some d-types have a standard contract they use with all s-types. Others will negotiate each contract individually.

If you or your partner(s) want a contract, remember to include ways to change the contract later. Relationships need room to grow and something always gets forgotten.

10.1.14 Handkerchief Codes

Handkerchief codes originated in the gay men's subculture of the 60s and 70s. It spread from there to kink. Not many people use handkerchief code any longer, if only because most of us find our partners online these days. Several different hankie code lists were published in books and magazines for gay men in the early 80s, and possibly earlier.

The code uses a combination of color and location. Left signals top/dom, right signals bottom/sub. The color indicated the activity.

If you want, you can look online for lists of hanky code color meanings. But be aware that, like any code system developed across a huge community that operated in secret, not all the lists will agree.

The hankie code was also sometimes called the flag code, and that's where you will most likely run into it in practice. Someone might say they 'flag' black to mean they are into S&M or 'flag' grey for bondage.

10.1.15 Topping from the Bottom

Topping from the bottom is a negative term for s-types and/or bottoms who try to control a scene. Note, again, the conflation of sub and bottom. This is a term you may hear as a criticism of an s-type or bottom. Sometimes it's a warning that they aren't a good person to scene with—that they are known to be manipulative. (see: Missing Stair) Sometimes it's used to criticize someone who begs a lot or is a bratty sub or... well, anything a given person may not like from an s-type or bottom they scene with. It may also be used within a scene, 'stop topping from the bottom.'

There are several potential issues with this term, which makes a lot of folks dislike it.

First, the implication that a bottom shouldn't have any say or control in a scene. Not all bottoms are s-types. If a scene doesn't involve D/s than the bottom has just as much control over the scene as the top.

Second, some bottoms are dominants. A dominant bottom damn well should be controlling the scene from the bottom. They are the dominant!

Third, everyone has different expectations and experiences. Some d-types see a sub begging or asking for something as 'topping from the bottom.' Others like hearing a sub begging or pleading for something.

I'm leery of this term because it feels like it short circuits communication. Better to say outright, 'I don't like to hear subs begging, take what I give your or scene with someone else.' Or 'they can be very manipulative, most of us avoid scening with them.' Or whatever you actually mean. But as always, YMMV.

10.1.16 The Old Guard

'The Old Guard' refers to kinksters (and the way kink was done) back before the internet. Scene legend sometimes speaks of the Old Guard as some original way kink communities functioned. A time when everyone followed the same protocol and rules. If you knew the secret handshake you could move across the country, visit the local kink enclave, and it would be exactly like home just with different people.

Thanks to FetLife, I've been lucky enough to know and learn from a few folks who've been kinky since before I was born and... well, it makes a pretty myth. Many kink groups were indeed hard to find and often leery of who they let in. But there was no one, unified 'Old Guard' approach to BDSM. There were some somewhat unified subcultures, the gay leather scene being the best known of these. But at best it was several different kinky subcultures that were somewhat related.

Unfortunately, being 'Old Guard' has a certain cachet in the Scene. Some folks try to gain some attention or respect by claiming to be Old Guard. Or by claiming they learned the secret traditions of the Old Guard.

Learn from the elders of the Scene. They have a lot to teach us. But (to invert a polyam saying), there are lots of wrong ways, but there is no one right way. Anyone trying to claim Old Guard credentials to push their version of twueism is best ignored.

10.1.17 The Submissive Has the Real Power

A common saying about power exchange that is somewhat controversial. It's meant as a reminder that the submissive is the one giving power to the d-type and can revoke that at any time and end the scene/relationship. But that ignores that the d-type can *also* end the scene/relationship at any time.

Basically, some folks seem to need the reminder that the s-type's consent is required and their giving (or revoking) consent gives them power in the scene. Which, yes they do, yes it does, any d-type who doesn't get this shouldn't be doing power exchange. But it ignores or erases the importance of the d-type's consent and, in some uses, makes it sound like the power the d-type has during the power exchange isn't real, that the submissive isn't *really* submitting, it's basically an elaborate role play.

Which... a lot of power exchange folks don't appreciate. The power the d-type has is real because the s-type gives it to them. That the s-type can take it back doesn't make it less real. And everyone has the 'power' to end stuff at any time because that's how consent works.

10.1.18 TNG

Okay, this one won't be unusual to nerds or polyam folk who live where there are a lot of polyamory groups.

TNG stands for The Next Generation. In practice, it means kinksters under 35. Almost exclusively used to designate a certain group or activity as having age restrictions for members or attendees.

10.1.19 Vanilla

'Vanilla' refers to non-kinky people and things. A person might be vanilla or someone might refer to vanilla sex.

Some folks in the Scene use vanilla as a derogatory term as if vanilla were bland or boring. But face it, vanilla is the most popular ice cream flavor for a reason. It's in every cookie and cake recipe for the same reason. Vanilla is awesome. And many kinky folks often include some vanilla in our lives. Anyone who is derogatory of vanilla is someone you probably don't want in your life. Remember YKINMK and that's okay—even if your kink is no kink.

10.1.20 WIITWD

Okay, quick and easy, 'WIITWD' is an abbreviation for 'what it is that we do.' As mentioned at the beginning of this book, setting a clear, concise and *complete* definition of BDSM or 'being kinky' isn't easy. WIITWD is a nice stand-in for when you want to be inclusive of all the random, fun, weirdness that goes on within the Scene.

It also functions as a noun, unlike 'being kinky,' which can make grammar easier.

10.2 Stuff that Can Be Confused with Kink

10.2.1 Hierarchical Relationships

Other types of hierarchical relationships can at first glance look like power exchange kink. Most of these are het-centric with the assumption that hierarchy is based on gender.

10.2.1.1 'Taken in Hand' and 'Christian Domestic Discipline'

I've heard a few kinksters, especially M/f master/slave folks, speak of feeling a connection with these. But their basic relationship premises and approaches are foreign to the precepts of kink. 'Taken in Hand' and 'Christian Domestic Discipline' are coming not from free choice and consent. Instead, they come from the assumption that men should have the power in their relationships and the right to discipline their wives.

Taken in Hand writings and discussions tend to promote the pseudoscientific idea of the 'alpha male.' TiH is slightly less gender-based than CDD. Some TiH folks will include relationships with an 'alpha female' and submissive male in their ranks. But for the most part, the existence of relationships with women in charge isn't acknowledged or welcomed.

Christian Domestic Discipline doesn't indulge in the 'alpha

male' pseudoscience. It is (as the name says) based in Christianity: God has ordained men as the head of household and women should submit to them.

Several other hierarchical relationship styles follow this general pattern.

10.2.1.2 FLR

FLR or 'female-led relationship' is a common term for... well, just that. Relationships with women in charge. Unlike the above stuff, FLR usually doesn't rely on a philosophy of gender essentialism, pseudoscience, or religious dictates. FLR relationships are chosen by the individuals involved. There's no idea that FLR is universally right or everyone should do FLR. Most FLR would fit in with kink communities and be welcome as D/s relationships. But they prefer doing their own thing. More power to them.

10.2.2 Hot Wife/Stag&Vixen

Hot-wifing is when a man gets off on his wife having sex with other people. Stag & Vixen is a variation on this that allows for the fun to go both ways. Both are types of ethical nonmonogamy.

I've seen people say that hot-wifing is a kink and others insisting that it isn't a kink. Regardless, most folks who explore this type of nonmonogamy aren't part of the Scene unless they have other kinks they are into.

Anyway, the relevant thing here isn't whether or not hot-wifing is kinky. The relevant thing is that hot-wifing can be confused with cucking. Hot-wifing, in all its variations, doesn't include the humiliation and shaming of the cuck that are embedded in cucking. Especially since both cucking and Stag&Vixen (and possibly hot-wifing in general) refer to the temporary sex partner as the 'bull.'

So if someone is looking for a 'bull' don't assume they are doing (or not doing) humiliation.

(My thanks to Secret Vixen for answering my questions about Stag & Vixen. You can learn more on her website: http://secretvixen.blog/.)

(No one ever asked my opinion, but you're reading my book so I assume you care. ;-) If anyone did ask me, I'd say that hotwife folks of all varieties should be welcome in the Scene. They've usually got a strong mix of voyeurism and exhibitionism going on. But like FLR folks, they are usually happy doing their own thing and (again) more power to 'em.)

Wrapping Up

So, that's it. I've said all I can think of on combining polyam and kink. Hopefully it's enough (possibly more than enough) to get your started.

Thank you for including me on your journey to explore kink and polyamory. I hope I've been helpful to you. As always, nothing works for everyone. Take what fits, leave what doesn't.

And don't forget to have fun together.

11 Kink List

1. Sensory Play: stuff that's all about the 'five' senses (in one way or another)

- Impact play: includes some kinds of pain play, but there are ways to do impact play that aren't painful

- Sensory Deprivation: removing one sense tends to enhance others

- Blindfolds

- Earplugs

- Full bodysuits

- Hoods

- Electro play: Some folks love using TENS units and other safe tools for applying electricity to the body

- Temperature play: Using ice, heating pads, sometimes fire (with proper safety precaution) on different parts of the body (usually erogenous zones)

- Pain play: stuff that's intended to be painful

2. Emotional Play

A. Control: can be part of a scene without invoking power exchange

- Breath Control: often considered edge play, using hands or tools to control someone's ability to breathe

- Gags: should be self-explanatory

- Mental bondage

B Humiliation

- Golden showers: peeing on someone/being peed on

- Cuckolding/Cuckqueening: one person in a committed relationship having another sex partner, with the intent to humiliate the cuck.

- Scat play: anything involving, well, human scat

- Verbal humiliation: the most common version is calling a sex partner insulting names during sex

- Sissy/sissification: 'feminizing' a man and/or 'turning them into a woman.' Highly problematic when played straight. however, many gender-nonconforming men and AMABs who think they might be trans have used it as a safe way to explore gender, gender-bending, etc.

C Fear: did you know that fear and arousal are closely related? Yeah.

- Gunplay: using a (usually fake) gun to stimulate fear in a scene

- Knife play: ditto

- Rape play: simulating rape (with full consent of all parties)

- Mindfucks: creating fear by making the bottom think something (usually very extreme) is happening when it isn't

D Invoking Taboos: the illicit is appealing, pretty straightforward.

- Teacher kinks: scenes where one person pretends to be a teacher/professor

- Religious kink: not much more taboo for some folks that mixing sex and religion. Of course, for other folks, it's Tuesday.

- Nazi kink: yeah, it's a thing. 'nuff said.

- Race kink: roleplay based on real-world racial disparity, historical or current. US chattel slavery is a popular 'setting.' Another problematic one, though I have heard one black woman say she used such scenes to work through her anger and pain re: racism in the real world. Basically: don't judge if you don't know the details, but often problematic as fuck.

3. Sexual: doing sex... differently

- Exhibitionism: liking being watched while you do sex

- Voyeurism: liking watching other people do sex

- Hot Wife or Vixen/Stag: Cucking without the humiliation aspect, the focus is on Exhibitionism and Voyeurism. If called Vixen/Stag may go both ways. Not always considered kinky.

- Chastity: no one to my knowledge has made a practical chastity belt for folks with vulvas (believe me, they've tried), but there are *many* chastity devices for keeping that penis locked down.

- Tease: you know the slur 'cock tease?' Yeah, some people like that. And several variations on, including stopping right before orgasm.

- Fisting: putting the whole hand (or in some cases an actual fist) in a vagina or anus

- Pegging: using a strap-on on someone

- Edging: related to teasing but more extreme. Every time someone gets close to coming, stimulation stops. Rinse/repeat for as long as desired, then end sex play—with or without allowing the orgasm. Related to orgasm denial.

- Orgasm denial: chastity in kink is when you are locked away and can't touch. Orgasm denial is when you are constantly aroused and not allowed to come. May incorporate teasing or edging.

- Repeated orgasms: being brought to orgasm repeatedly in a short space of time. At a point, will become painful.

- Come on command: training/being trained to come on command

- Sounding: inserting something (usually a thin metal rod) into the urethra

4. Other

- Hypnosis: using hypnosis in a scene

- Roleplay: taking on roles for a scene—cheerleader, firefighter, stewardess inducting someone into the mile high club—because the role play adds to the fun

- Body modification: ranges from piercings to tattoos to... more extreme stuff. Generally considered edgeplay.

Also By Jess Mahler

Polyamory on Purpose Guides

Polyamory and Pregnancy
The Polyamorous Home
Safer Sex for the Non-Monogamous

Fiction

The Bargain
Whips & Fangs

Upcoming Books

The next Polyamory on Purpose guide:
Abuse in Polyamory
Will be out July 2021.
Jess Mahler's next fiction novel
Planting Life in a Dying City
Will be out January 2021.
Become a Patron for early access.

About Jess Mahler

Jess has never been one to do things the 'easy' way. Which is probably why she spent several years pulling together a family-of-choice from across the country. The family, including a demon, a dragon, and a cat, hopes to settle in the Appalachians where Jess' heart has been rooted for as long as she can remember.

Health issues keep her from taking a more active role in *tikkun olam*, repairing the world, so she writes to spread knowledge and ideas. Her fiction and non-fiction both explore different ways of living and being.

Jess has 15 years in polyam relationships including dealing with legal challenges, abusive relationships, group living, LDRs, and a good bit more. As an autistic autodidact, you never know when she'll pull an odd bit of knowledge out of her back pocket that gives a new perspective on an old problem.

Copyright

Polyamory and Kink

by Jess Mahler

Paperback version | Copyright 2020 Jess Mahler

http://jessmahler.com

www.ingramcontent.com/pod-product-compliance
Lightning Source LLC
Chambersburg PA
CBHW031235250726
48655CB00005B/1960